Copyright information

Dedication

To every depression warrior who has ever journeyed through the darkness.

May you find compassion, love and understanding on your journey.

Acknowledgements

Special thanks to; Karen Pickett, Talis Kimberley, Simon Fairbourn, Timothy Yarham, Jani Franck, Clare Dacosta-Funkhauser, Mark Edgar and Cat Treadwell for a vast assortment of inspiration, cheer-leading, conceptual deciphering, encouragement, But more than anything, for believing in me and helping to make this book a reality. My gratitude to you guys specifically is unending, without you, I would have given up before I had finished even the first paragraph.

Special thanks go to my Indiegogo contributors, especially to the following:

Jani Franck

Janet Tahiri

Timothy Yarham

Tim Earthey

Ricky Gellisen

Jane Goldsack

Andrea Parker

…as well as all my other lovely contributors who enabled me to get this book in print.

Introduction

"Depression is a common mental disorder. Globally, more than 350 million people of all ages suffer from depression."
[World Health Organisation Fact sheet N°369, October 2012]

I would like my introduction to this book to be two-fold as there are messages, stories and feelings included within this book that are for two very different kinds of reader. Firstly the people who are dealing with depression but also the loved ones of people who have depression. I will address you separately for the purposes of introduction only. From the first chapter onwards, you will both receive the same words.

Please note that any parts of this book which are written in **bold** type are entries taken directly, unedited from my personal journal shared in these pages for illustrative purposes in the hopes I can shed some light on the world inside the mind of a depressed person. Anything written in *italic* is a recollection of that time. I hope that by separating things in this way it will help you to understand the differences in perception.

Dear People who are dealing with depression,

Hi,

I am Alexis, it is good to meet you. In the following pages I will be telling my story as well as giving suggestions for how people who are not walking in the darkness can help and support you during your journey with depressive illness. It will be hard to read in places. There are some parts which may well be triggers for you. I ask you with all the love in the world to ensure that you are "safe" before reading the parts I have distinctly marked as "triggering". There is absolutely no shame in not reading them. In fact, I ask you here and now to consider your mental state at all times. Feel free to read only bits, or read all of it. I leave that down to your judgement.

I want to take a moment with you, dear reader to tell you something. You are not alone. There are at least 350 million of us out there who have walked in the darkness that depression has thrown around us. I know it can feel as though nobody cares. But I care and your family cares, however much the illness tries to convince you otherwise. Over the following few chapters I will be bearing my soul in your honour. I'm not writing this book to be dramatic, nor for recognition. I wrote this book for YOU. I wrote it because when I was walking in the shroud of depression I was unable to find the words to tell my loved ones what was going on inside, to explain to them what I was feeling/thinking and how they could help me.

If you too are struggling with that...I suggest grabbing a post it note, or an old envelope; something you can use as a page marker...find the appropriate chapter, mark it and give this book to your loved one, have them read my story and perhaps it will help them to relate that to what you are going through. I am more than happy to share my experiences and my story on your behalf, in the hope that I can help to be a voice when you feel you need someone to speak the words you are struggling to find.

Never forget that you are cared for, hang in there because brighter skies will come. It may be a while and the journey will be hard, but there is ALWAYS hope. Hold on to that hope tightly and stay strong.

My love, hope and hugs always,

Alexis

Dear loved ones of depression sufferers,

It can be incredibly hard to live with someone who has a depressive illness. There are times when the reality in which you are living and the world inside your loved ones head are two VERY different places. It can be hard to know whether you are doing the right things, saying the right things, interpreting your loved ones behaviour rightly or wrongly. That is why I wrote this book.

During my deepest bout of depressive illness I tore apart my family. I did not feel capable of expressing my inner turmoil to the world and so I behaved badly and pushed them away until they were forced to make the most difficult decision of all; their sanity or my presence in their home. In the end, they chose their sanity, a decision for which I am ever grateful to them for making.

In hindsight it was the kindest, most love-filled decision they could have made. But it was not an easy one. At the time I was hurt and angry; I didn't understand that it was my behaviour which had caused such a horrific mess. I respect my foster-mum so very much for having the courage to stand up and tell me outright that it was too much for them to handle. But most of all I respect her for continuing to support my journey through life and loving me even after all I have put my family through. Now that I have found my path back to sanity, I can see that it must have torn her apart to ask that of me. I hope that the words, personal stories and ideas in the following pages are of some value to you, that you may find some comfort and understanding among these pages and that subsequently you may never find yourself in the position I put my family in.

All I ask of you is that you read the following chapters with an open mind and a non-judgemental heart. May you find clarity, explanation and love in this book. Alexis xx

What IS depression?

According to the British medical association "Illustrated medical dictionary" (2013 edition), depression is:

"Feelings of sadness, hopelessness, and a loss of interest in life, combined with a sense of reduced emotional wellbeing. Symptoms may vary with the severity of the depression."

What does that mean in reality for sufferers?

Depression is the term given to a range of symptoms which, when experienced together affect a person's mood, concentration and ability to maintain their usual routine and way of life. These symptoms generally last anything between weeks, months or even in some cases years and results in the person suffering from extended periods of low mood and potentially experiencing feelings of self-loathing, self-harm or suicidal thoughts and or feelings.

The symptoms are wide-ranging and different for everyone. My own experiences of depression tend to result in the following symptoms (this is from my own personal journal, thus grammatical errors/ spelling mistakes are not edited out):

" food and drink:

little chance I'll eat anything. If it requires more than one mouthful, don't even bother. usual staple diet in depressive mode for me is chicken, chocolate and ice cream. have been known to go days without feeling hungry or up to eating.

Drink is mostly normal. [note: I do not generally drink alcohol, apart from special occasions]

sleep:

A couple of hours most nights. Absolutely none others, followed by extreme sleeping once my body hits empty. Uncontrollable.

socialising:

As little as possible. When at my lowest I will hibernate for extreme periods. Absolutely do not want to be around people. It means they either pity you, make allowances for you or feel bad for not helping. Worst of all is reflective

guilt: they feel guilty for being ok, while I feel guilty for making them feel bad.

Working:

Either extremely hyperactive overcompensation for crap mood, or totally useless and lack concentration.

Self injury:

Extremely variable. The more unwell I get, the greater the likelihood of cutting myself becomes.

Suicidal feelings/ thoughts/ self-loathing:

General feelings of self-loathing reach a peak during depressive cycles, unable to see any good or worth in myself. Suicidal only in extreme depressive mode. Thankfully rare.

Sex drive:

Tends to go between one of two settings; insatiable and non-existent. (both much moreso than is "normal" for me)

Other:

Generally for me the first sign is that the house is a pigsty and I have absolutely detached, barely notice until I run out of crockery or clothes. Little or no inclination to sort it out and cannot even begin to remember why it is so messy.

Personal hygiene also goes out the window. Mostly because my brain is in hyper drive worrying about absolutely everything in ridiculous detail and it runs out of energy."

Please note, this is NOT an exhaustive list of symptoms, it is merely the ones that I experience most regularly when I am feeling depressed. Most of these are covered in much greater depth throughout the following chapters.

Diagnosis

Imagine for just a moment that you have never read a map before, but suddenly you are asked to read a map which has no markings or hints for how you should get from A to B All of a sudden there is a reason for your feelings and illness, but it is one of which you have little understanding and there is suddenly a whole new terminology which can at best be confusing and at worst terrifying. The road stretches off into a distance that you cannot begin to comprehend, let alone plan for, and each step is a whole new terrain full of different monsters; monsters who know just how to tear you to shreds. That is how it can feel when you are first given a diagnosis of a depressive illness.

It is a daunting and often self-stigmatised situation to find yourself in and those early days are often tinged with fear that you are going insane. This is not the case of course; there is merely a discrepancy between the chemicals inside the brain which is causing you to feel unwell.

Most GPs these days have a pretty good understanding of mental health issues and are reasonably good at diagnosing illnesses such as depression. Such diagnosis is not always easy because seeking the help you need feels entirely counterproductive to a person experiencing the lows of depression. This is because the illness knows that if you seek help then you will no longer be in the throes of the self-hating, self-doubting fits that the illness is so very good at putting you into.

Access to professional mental health treatment (in the UK) can sometimes take weeks depending on how busy your local mental health team is, which is in my opinion absolutely disgusting. The help is available; however, it is a waiting game between initial diagnosis and access to the counselling or psychiatric consultations.

I remember well those first few months after being diagnosed. Suddenly I was a person who had a diagnosis of mental illness, one of which I had little understanding and one which left too much shock, fear and desolation to have the courage to get the answers that would have helped me understand.   Obviously time and society has moved on a lot in the ten years since I was first diagnosed, but now, just like then you get good doctors and you get bad ones. A good doctor will take the time to listen and help you to understand this strange new land which you are walking in.

One thing I would suggest is that if your loved one is as scared and incapable of asking the questions themselves as I was, then you as their advocate could really help them by being the one to ask those important questions which will help them to understand; questions such as "what are the possible side effects of this medication? Are there any helpful services locally that can provide some support? Where can I get more information? What are the current waiting times like for access to specialists? (if required) these are the questions we often need answered but are too busy trying to understand to think to ask at the time. Make sure that you understand their answers, even if your loved one does not as they may well ask you later what the professional said or to explain it in more understandable terms.

You see, the most difficult thing about dealing with healthcare professionals is that they are under-resourced and oversubscribed and thus do not always realise that the brevity of their answers is not actually helpful to someone newly diagnosed with depression who is struggling to understand this big, scary word that they have now been given as a diagnosis.

My personal favourite phrase for the best doctor I ever had was "ok, please tell me that again in layman's terms, I'm sorry but I'm afraid I don't speak doctorese" and she would smile, apologise for not being clear then helpfully explain it to me in more simple terms.

It took me a number of years to find a doctor who understood mental health on a level much deeper than "The medical dictionary says x, y, and z". She offered many options and would take the time to explain things, then ask what I felt would help. This was, in my opinion, a very helpful and worthwhile exercise, as at the very least it helped me to feel like I had some control over the situation. This can be an extremely stressful and worrying time for the person who is going through the diagnostic process as well as for family members and it is totally understandable to feel afraid, confused and shocked. There are numerous useful sources of information out there; a quick search on the internet should provide details of a service local to you.

The following is an extract from a journal entry I wrote a number of years ago (Circa 2004/5) about receiving my own diagnosis and how it felt.

"That first moment I saw her, she was stood before me, with an expression matching mine, fear-filled, confused and almost apathetic to the world which surrounded us. Surrounded, enveloped yet crushed us both. From this moment forward we would be forced to live as one, forced to share our every waking moment and every now shattered dream with one another, neither of us had been informed if there was a loophole, a little-known way to step out of the living hell that was to come, so we stood together, yet alone, so very alone in this room, this moment, this desolation.

There was a fear in her eyes which I only half recognised. That same look of confused fear you see right before the car smashes the rabbit's skull as you obliterate it into its new state of road kill. That same terrified smile that says "please don't ask" that self same stomach-churning moment where you watch the world fall from beneath your feet and realise that actually you forgot how to care, how to connect with the emotional side of yourself.

We stood facing one another for a long moment, our hands touching through the cold, glass that separated my reflection from my real self. You see, only half an hour before this moment, I had been living a perfectly "normal" life, a life which raged between sudden self-hatred and albeit rare moments of self-love. But I had been normal, hadn't I? I had stood among my peers as the emo kid, the semi-goth who had few friends but didn't really care for people much anyway.

But now? NOW I had a label, now I had a word for this monster that stared back from the mirrors cool, shiny surface. She was called Depression, she was both inside and external to me, we were intrinsically linked by the sharing of blood, skin, tears, bones and brains.

Depression? Who on earth was she? How did she get inside me? How did this union occur? Why must we now live as one? What did or didn't I do that now forced us to become one with each other? Suddenly a thousand questions sprang to mind, how could my life change to this overnight?

So there we stood, my reflection and I, staring at one another through a mirror. Locked together in a battle-dance of unknown length. Neither of us will ever win over the other, but we will forever be holding one another hostage for a while. Gagging either the positive or the negative. The fight continues......"

It was a very scary time in my life, being 20 years old and suddenly having a diagnosis of depression. I had a very limited support network back then and wouldn't have had the first clue where to turn for help. Thankfully my boss at the time was very understanding and helped me to realise that the whole situation really wasn't as frightening as it seemed and helped me to come to terms with the illness.

Medication

In Western medicine there are two main treatments for depressive illnesses. These are medication and counselling. Obviously everyone responds differently to the different regimes of treatment and there is, therefore no "norm" of treatment. I would like to share with you in this chapter a little advice which I have honed over the years from personal experience.

If you (or a loved one) are prescribed medication for depression, then it is important that you continue taking that medication until you are told to stop by a medical professional. It is perfectly normal for a depressed person to feel as though the medication isn't doing anything for the first four to six weeks of being on a new medication regime, this is because your body is still adjusting the levels of serotonin in the brain and it takes a while to register that it has changed. On the flipside of this, it is all too easy, once the medication has begun working to feel as though you are miraculously healed and therefore no longer need the tablets. This is absolutely not the case and stopping them suddenly without lowering the dosage under medical supervision can prove dangerous. It can also result in the symptoms worsening and the person feeling much worse than they did even before medication.

Often people who are on medication for a depressive illness feel resentful of needing a medicine in order to live a normal life, but it is important to remember that there is absolutely no shame in needing something to help balance the levels of serotonin in the brain. If you friend or loved one is struggling to come to terms with the necessity of medication, I would suggest explaining to them that there is no shame involved, remind them that it is perfectly normal for someone who has a broken leg to seek the appropriate treatment and that antidepressant medication is really no big deal. This may help the person not to feel so ashamed or stupid about needing their medication. A little girl of my acquaintance once said to me "You need your medication in the same way that I need Insulin. So just imagine your brain has diabetes if that will help", she's not such a little girl now, but her wise words have stuck with me ever since.

It is also important for the friends and loved ones of a person who has a mental illness to remember that the first drug that is offered is not always going to be the one that works for the person. Most of the people with a depressive illness I have spoken with have tried several drugs before they found the one which works best for them, this is because everyone is different and what may work well for one person may well be wrong for someone else. Encouragement and support will really help your friend or loved one to find the right regime for their needs. It can be incredibly difficult going through the medication lottery phase of treatment, but once the right regime is found, life becomes much easier to cope with and an awful lot less scary for all involved.

Often what really helps a person is a mixture of counselling and medication. Seeking talk therapies can be excruciatingly difficult because it feels as though you are some kind of freak for needing someone to talk to, even though you are (perhaps) surrounded by people with whom you feel you should be able to communicate your feelings. Rest assured, if your loved one is seeking counselling, this is a VERY positive step. In my experience that fog of emotions which is typical of depressive illness makes it very difficult for you to discuss things with the people you love, for fear of causing them to hurt or be upset because you are angry at the world and the very last thing you want is to tell someone you love how messed up that world inside your brain is. Talking to a therapist allows a brutal honesty uncharacteristic of most human relationships, where you do not have to worry that you may not express yourself in a socially acceptable way, but instead you are free to vent out whatever is going on inside. I would even go so far as to say that a friend or loved one of a person who has depression should actively encourage their loved one to seek counselling, as it offers a level of release which you cannot find elsewhere.

One other thing I would like to mention here (while on the subject of talk therapies) is help lines. I want to take a moment to dispel the myth that there is any shame whatsoever in calling them. It is their job to listen and allow a person who is in mental distress to voice their feelings without any form of judgement. I was discussing this book with a friend the other day who told me that he has on numerous occasions used such help lines and has always found them to be useful services for those moments of darkness when talking to a loved one is out of the question. It is my suggestion that you offer the telephone number of such organisations as are available in your area to your loved one, you never know when they will come in handy.

Some people find that alternative therapies such as reiki, meditation, aromatherapy and acupuncture can be useful in relieving the symptoms of depressive illness. In my experience alternative therapies such as meditation and reiki have been very useful tools in my arsenal against depression.

Meditation allows you to transport yourself to a "calm space" for a while without ever having to leave your room. This can give you the opportunity to step away from the things which are causing you stress for a while and recharge your internal batteries.

First firmly affix your own oxygen mask

I would like to offer a little sanity retaining advice for the loved ones of someone living with depression, as this is the main inspiration behind this book. During the months when I was in my worst bout of depression I drove my loved ones, most noticeably my foster-mum to distraction as my unreliability, inability to keep promises and general unpredictable behaviour put immense amounts of pressure on them. The pressure got greater and greater as I lost touch with the reality of the situation, but so did my oblivion as to how my behaviour was affecting those around me.

Unfortunately, it is often the case that depressed person is unable to see that their behaviour/ needs are putting strain on other people. It is like being in an invisible bubble where you can touch, see and hear the outside world but you cannot particularly understand the subtleties of it. At no point did it ever even occur to me that I was behaving in a manner which was totally different from how I believed I was being. The truth is the depressed person is living inside their own head.

Whether you take a step back to breathe or not is somewhat irrelevant, but what help can you offer if you are running on empty yourself? While everyone can run on empty to some degree and still cope, it is harder when you are trying to support someone whose needs and behaviours are so unpredictable that they begin to send you into a place of mental discomfort yourself. Your loved one would, if they were thinking clearly want you to take whatever space you need as well as supporting them; nobody wants other people to make themselves ill on their behalf.

My most memorable experience of this was at the psychiatric assessment. I had asked my foster-foster- mum to come with me because I truly believed I would be hospitalised as I was suicidal at this point, but also terrified of what may or may not come next. During the consultation I was doing the best I could to reach out to the CPN [community psychiatric nurse], but in all honesty I was struggling to understand the protocols of the situation I was in. I knew I needed help, but I wasn't at all sure how to get access to it. We talked for almost an hour then all hell broke loose. I think the following blog entry from the night in question explains why someone who is supporting a friend or loved one who has a depressive illness needs to take time and space from the person in order to maintain their own sanity before trying to give help and support to their loved one.

"It has been a long and difficult day. Emotional on a very heavy level. Today I went to the psychiatrist for the first time. My foster- mum

came with me and we talked to the psychiatrist together. It was hard to hear how much my behaviour is tearing apart her family. Tearing apart the only people I have that I can call family.

Hardest of all was hearing this woman, who loved and accepted me into her heart is now ripping herself to shreds with guilt that she cannot save me. She cannot be my hero this time.

What she doesn't realise, what she cannot bring herself to accept is that she was my hero that moment I first heard her sing. She was my hero when she brought me here. She IS my hero now; she always will be my hero, no matter what comes next.

The truth is...A hero isn't someone who saves you. A true hero is someone who loves you enough to stand beside you in those darkest hours and dares to trust you enough to let you save YOURSELF. Especially when doing so hurts them to watch. THAT is bravery and courage...and mum...you have buckets of both. You admitted the truth, you cannot be the one to save me and I thank you, truly for your honesty. It hurts, it's hard to hear, but it is an act of love to know when you must save yourself rather than letting someone tear you apart, albeit without intentionally doing so.

She did the best a mother could. She loved me enough to give me a chance. Albeit a chance that I blew by putting her in this position. The fact of the matter is, even if she were the superhero that she longs to be, she STILL couldn't save me. Nobody can, the only one capable of saving me right now, is me. I only wish I knew how I am supposed to do that.

So this one goes out to you, mum.

My hero. My friend and My inspiration always, no matter what comes next, know that you will ALWAYS be my hero. I love you."

Looking back on that entry, I am very much aware of the cathartic effects that day had over the entire period of my life. It was the line in the sand which signifies the beginning of my recovery. In hindsight I was looking for someone else to fix my issues, until the point where it was stated blatantly and without subtlety that there was no quick fix for someone in my situation. This entry was important to share with you because I think it outlines how painful the situation can become between two people who care for one another deeply, when one is unable to help the other during a difficult period in their life.

My advice to anyone put in the position my foster-mum was in; the main supporter role of a friend or loved one who has a depressive illness is really quite simple. Give as much support as you are able, but don't be afraid to step back in those moments when things get too much. It is important that you are coping before you try to support the friend or loved one who has a depressive illness; otherwise you will make the situation worse and more complex for both of you.

I would suggest talking to them gently and explaining that you need a little headspace and that you love them no matter what, but right now you need to take a step back because you are feeling overwhelmed. This means they are not left questioning your thoughts and feelings towards them and will cause less stress to all involved than if you suddenly vanish from their support space without a word. That just leaves them questioning themselves as to what they did wrong, whether you still care about them and if you will ever come back.

Another suggestion is to try not to be the sole source of support, where possible try to ensure that the person has a whole raft of people around them so that each gets a break from being the supporter and has time and space to recharge their batteries without leaving the friend or loved one who has a depressive illness feeling alone. This will make life easier for both the depressed person and the people around them as it means that they have more than one shoulder to cry on if you are unavailable. It also means that they are more able to maintain relationships in a healthier and less-detrimental way for everyone involved.

Encourage social interaction where possible, but be aware that they may not feel up to seeing or talking to people as often as a non-depressed person is. This is one of the many side effects of the illness and is truly no reflection on anyone.

It is important to understand that when the veils of depression fall upon someone, it is very difficult for them to see beyond the private prison inside of their head. Therefore, understanding that they are putting pressure on other people by not coping with daily life in a reasonable way, is like trying to describe the colour of air. Your loved one is not intentionally putting stress and strain on you, they are simply incapable of seeing the world outside of themselves clearly enough to relate to it on a level where they can see how their behaviour affects you or anyone else. Try to be patient but ensure that you have your own oxygen mask firmly affixed before you attempt to help someone else with theirs, it's a tough situation to be in, but it does have its rewarding moments too.

Capturing the brain weasels

Brain weasels is the name I give to those nasty little self hating thoughts that boom around inside one's head until they seem utterly reasonable. Some examples of these are "you're not good enough" "they are all laughing at you" "nobody really likes you" but in terms of depression they are much more likely to stick around and set up a little encampment in your head. I would describe them as being like an army of little weasels with tiny black paintbrushes which take any positive, happy thoughts or feelings and immediately paint them black. Unfortunately, these brain weasels are very good at finding new and innovative ways of making any achievements seem utterly insignificant in relation to anything that anyone else has done. There have been many times when the weasels have decided it's party time, most noticeably in those moments when one is not feeling particularly good about things and suddenly the tiniest thing can convince you that you have failed, no matter how incredible your achievements may have seemed to the outside world.

One example of this was at a party I attended. I was feeling particularly uncomfortable at this particular party due to some people I didn't particularly want to talk to being there, when a close friend made a joke about my cooking (I am, in all sincerity a notoriously bad cook) but my friend jokingly passed comment on it in front of a small group of mutual friends. Immediately, I felt utterly useless and was convinced within seconds that it was some kind of euphemism for "Lexi is useless at everything and we only want her in the group as a source of amusement. She's too stupid to ever be truly accepted by us as an equal." now on a good day, I would have simply threatened to cook her dinner or something else jovial, however on this occasion I was already being subjected to the brain weasel hate speech, so this comment was suddenly an unequivocal confirmation that I was utterly worthless. That night I cried myself to sleep, fearing that everyone believed me to be stupid and worthless and I withdrew my friendship from said friend for a good few months before I was at a point mentally where I was able to express to her that her comments had really wobbled my self esteem. After we talked things through it became apparent that it was just a flippant comment which I had totally overreacted to because of my mental state at the time. We are now friends again and both much more aware of one another's feelings/emotional states.

Once the weasels have decided to throw a party, it can be very difficult to ignore them. Anything which holds even a hint of positivity can become an immediate trigger for them to remind you that you are absolutely useless. At this point it can be extremely difficult for you to take on board any kind of compliment, positive affirmation or supportive comment as they simply shoot it down as being a case of the person just wanting to shut you up.

My suggestion for dealing with someone who is at this point in the cycle is to accept that sometimes there just are no words which are capable of bringing comfort. What you can do, is be gentle with the person and try not to exacerbate the feelings of isolation and self-loathing. I would say the simplest way of doing this is to ensure that you are not overly or jovially critical of the person when you are aware that they are feeling vulnerable already. We all have weaknesses, but when one is the solitary performer at a brain weasel party, it can be extremely difficult to see that a personal joke is anything less than confirmation of your apparent worthlessness and an immediate source of humiliation which will often result in a depressed person replying with an uncalled-for level of reaction to something tiny and flippant.

Another point I would like to make here is that from a depressive point of view, it can be very difficult to brush off negative comments made about you, even many years later.

During bouts of depression there are often situations which I find to be triggering for anxiety and feelings of self-loathing. Over the last few years I have had several rounds of counselling, but one of the things I learned was particularly helpful for me was the chart I am about to share with you. It is one of the simplest ways to stop, take a step back and think about the truth of the situation and whether it is, in fact a situation which you are superimposing negative thoughts and feelings upon.

Take for example the situation above, I immediately believed myself to be a terrible person based upon one flyaway comment. My lack of self-worth fuelled the flames which served only to make me feel much worse than was truly necessary, when these situations arise I find it particularly useful to call upon the technique I learned on a depression related self-help course. There is a form (various versions of the one below exist, but this is my preferred version as it has a reminder at the bottom of what goes where) It is really beneficial for helping to rationalise those thoughts and emotions which can be so overpowering in the moment.

CBT Thought Record

Situation	Moods	Automatic Thoughts	Evidence for the Hot Thought	Evidence against the Hot Thought	Alternative Thoughts	Moods Now
Who was I with? What was I doing? When? Where?	Describe each mood you felt at the time in one word. Rate 0-100	What went though my mind just before I felt like this? What does this say about me, my life, the future? What am I afraid might happen? What is the worst that could happen? Any images or memories?	Circle Hot Thought in previous column. Evidence supporting the conclusion. Avoid mind reading or interpretation.	What evidence can you think of that does not support your hot thought.	Any alternative thoughts? Rate how much you believe each one 0-100.	For each mood rate, 0-100, how much you feel it now.

(Image sourced from http://cdn.ohsheglows.com/wp-content/uploads/2011/11/thought.jpg)

This technique specifically can be invaluable for helping a person to stop, take a step back and look at the situation with a little more clarity, as well as finding ways to move forward in a healthier mindset. These kinds of cognitive behavioural therapy (CBT) techniques can really help the person to understand that it is a reaction to an automatically negative self-view or thought which is making them feel bad about something and therefore take a step back from the situation and process what has happened in order to understand both the trigger, the situation and the most appropriate way to move forward and deal with the situation next time it arises. While this doesn't stop the thoughts, it can be beneficial in helping a depressed person to stop going around in circles by teaching them to disprove the thought without making a big deal about it.

Trust and autonomy

When wrapped in the dark veils of depression things inevitably seem negative and no matter what happens around you, you are incapable of seeing the positives from that dark place, thus making decisions can be incredibly difficult and energy burning at times, more-so than for a person who is not battling a mental illness.

When I was at my worst, it was very hard for me to listen to loved ones opinions about my behaviour or decisions; I felt as though they were criticising constantly, though in reality they were simply trying to help me see things with a little more clarity. The important thing here is that you know that the depressed person is not intentionally trying your patience; it is simply that they are living in a brain-chemically-adapted environment where their relationship with reality doesn't really make much sense and even when there are brief interludes of lucidity they probably haven't got the energy to be enthused about things anyway. The key to this is learning to tell the difference between their lucid days and days where the cloak of blackness has fallen. Try to catch them on a good day in order to have serious or emotionally charged conversations with them, otherwise you may well be discussing things with a person who isn't capable of taking things at face value and will take offence so easily that your conversation will inevitably end in tears, likely yours from frustration.

There are times when a depressed person just needs to vent about a situation or problem, without really wanting you to tell them the answer. Even if it appears quite straightforward to you, it might take them a little longer to see the obvious path among the more obscure, dangerous paths that seem to beckon them. To this day, I often call my foster-mum just to talk about random things so that I can clear some of the layers of rubbish out of my brain and find my own way through whatever situation I happen to be going through at the time.

It is important to me that I maintain my own independence and autonomy, but also sometimes knowing that she is someone who understands me and has seen me at my worst, means that I can trust her to tell me outright if she feels that I am in a bad headspace and therefore not making rational decisions. It is like having a safety net; that doesn't by any means mean that we don't have perfectly normal conversations too; it just means that we are both aware that this is one of my many coping mechanisms. It also does not mean that I am incapable of living a totally independent, normal life. It is just that sometimes a person with depression needs a little more support with organising their thoughts into an appropriate order to enable them to make a rational decision.

The fact is, if a friend or loved one who has a depressive illness is talking to you openly about their mental health then that means that you have reached the status of trusted person and should feel honoured that they feel comfortable enough in entrusting you with something so deeply personal and potentially soul-destroying.

People who have mental illnesses are stigmatised by society, this means that it is more difficult for us to speak openly about our mental illness, especially to people with whom we are not particularly familiar, such as co-workers, bosses even as far as healthcare professionals.

It is very difficult to show someone a mental illness; it is not obvious like a broken arm or leg. It is however just as serious. This is why it may well be very important for your loved one to have your support when seeking professional help with the illness. I will be covering advocacy in more depth in a later chapter.

Remember, your loved one is still the same person they always were, it's just that right now they are wrapped in a cloak of darkness which feels like it an unending whirlpool of pain, fear and dissociation from those whom they love.

There are times when you will need to be firm or blunt with your friend or loved one who has a depressive illness, telling them straight out how a situation is because under that cloak of blackness, subtlety is lost amidst the confusion of trying to decipher what is real and what is a superimposed alternate version of reality put in place by the depression. There were many times when the subtlety of human communication was lost to me in my darkest hours. Someone would do something kind. For example a neighbour offered me dinner one evening and I became too caught up in the veils of trying to work out if it was because they felt sorry for me or if it was some kind of way to keep an eye on me. I turned down all offers of help because they didn't fit inside my worldview, which was at that point that everyone hated, pitied or was afraid of me. I would sit alone in my room for long periods, trying hard to work out what things meant and instead of accepting help as I should have done, I would hide and exacerbate the situation out of fear and self-loathing.

Also, don't feel as though you cannot also seek support from your friend or loved one who has a friend or loved one who has a depressive illness, it can actually help them to feel like they are doing something constructive and give them a purpose if you allow them to also take on the role of supporter sometimes. It can remind them that they are not the only person on the planet who has "issues". Depression can be an incredibly isolating illness and leave them feeling as though they are somehow broken or their internal settings are stuck on overloaded.

When all is said and done it is important to remember that while friends and loved ones of people who are living with a depressive illness can be a support to their loved one, they cannot live their life for them. There will be times when the depressed person will need help and encouragement in order to make healthy decisions for themselves, but nobody can force them to make good choices.

What to say/not/why at different points in the cycle

For the most part a friend or loved one who has a depressive illness is a regular person, just like you. However, at times the brain weasels will take control of the person's brain and manipulate every word, action or situation and turn them into something entirely different from what a person who does not have a depressive illness perceives.

Thus, a perfectly simple conversation can suddenly feel like a war for no apparent reason at all. This is not because your friend or loved one who has a depressive illness is intent upon taking everything you do or say negatively. It is in fact because the deep dark mists of depression obscure a person's worldview in terms of love, trust and understanding. It is incredibly difficult in that dark place to understand the subtleties of interaction. I will try to explain some of these things in the rest of this chapter and offer as much explanation as possible from personal experience to give you some insight into why and how those things feel for someone who has depression.

No comments about a depressed person's appearance:

During the moments when the darkness has thrown its veil upon a person, it can be difficult to handle any kind of compliment. Any comments aimed at a depressed person's appearance will feel as though you are either mocking them, or just saying nice things because it is polite. I would suggest that a person who is very depressed is unlikely to have been taking pride in their appearance and may well have personal hygiene issues, it is likely that they are aware of it, vaguely but are unable to muster the energy to deal with it as well as dealing with the stresses and strains of everyday life which are magnified by a depressive illness.

Avoid being subtle

Avoid being subtle in your interactions with a depressed person. Their brain weasels are likely keeping their mind too cluttered for them to be able to decipher whether you are inferring something or not. Be blunt, in a kind way if possible, but don't leave things open to interpretation. At many points in a depressive cycle there are numerous pitfalls relating to communication, subtlety is one of them. Make life easier for both yourself and your friend or loved one by trying not to be subtle about things which are unnecessary. I would certainly rather you hurt me momentarily with your bluntness than spend hours questioning whether you meant what you thought you had made clear or something entirely different that my brain weasels have twisted your ambiguousness into.

(Brain weasels can convince you that black is white and vice versa. Don't make it easy for them to twist your words.) Simple things like this can avoid making life difficult for you and your loved ones.

Ensuring that your loved one has understood what you have said is an invaluable tool in fighting depressive illness. Ambiguity is one of depressions main fuels for making a bad situation worse. So long as the depressed person understands what has been said to them or how and why a situation is happening as it is, they will be better able to take on board your comments or actions and will be much more capable of responding in an appropriate and more constructive way.

Give simple instructions

When the brain weasels are throwing a grand ball with someone's brain as the main dance arena, it is incredibly difficult for them to decipher long and complex situations, instructions, lists or terminologies. Therefore what really is helpful is if you don't make a task sound bigger and scarier than it already is. Bearing in mind that at times something as simple as eating a bowl of cereal can be a mammoth task when depression has hit, then it is easy to realise that any task can be incredibly difficult, especially if it is given in such a way that the person cannot begin to decipher it from your instructions, let alone understand how it relates to them. So my advice here is to keep it simple.

Don't overcomplicate things and accept that they may well take longer to achieve said task than when they are fully present mentally. They are not being slow to annoy you, or because they don't *want* to do it, they are being slow because the brain is taking longer to access the energy and understanding reserves which enable them to do said thing. When I am in depressive mode I find it surprisingly difficult to complete a task if it is given in confusing or long-winded terms. If I am struggling to relate to a task, then it is likely that I will not even begin to attempt it because I am too caught up in the trying to understand headspace to be able to successfully achieve any kind of satisfactory result. Make life easier on both of you by giving clear, concise and simple directions, but try not to be patronising about it.

Also situations like doctor's appointments can be very stressful for someone who is battling a depressive illness, if such a situation is causing your friend or loved one to be anxious, try running through what will be expected of them during the consultation a few days before, this will help to allay some of the fears and stressors which come up from these kinds of situation.

Try not to put a depressed person down, even jokingly

When a depressed person is struggling to contain brain weasels they are already at a place inside where they are less capable of seeing anything positive or even remotely good about themselves, in fact all those things they usually love about you are probably annoying the hell out of them right now. This is the illness speaking and it is part of the cycle, the illness does not want a depressed person to have friends or loved ones who they can trust, because trust is one of the things that can really help the recovery process.

Where usually the depressed person is capable of taking a joke in general, there are some points in the depressive cycle where they are utterly unable to take any criticism at all, however jovial it may seem to the person outside of that head-space because it makes them feel as though those negative automatic thoughts that they are already fighting now have a cheerleader in the real world. This means they will find it all the more difficult to dismiss the brain weasel and will probably react to you in an overblown, argumentative way because you now symbolise the very things they are trying so hard to fight right now. It is best to think of that person right now as someone who is feeling incredibly vulnerable and is likely to take offence rather than being capable of laughing things off in the way that a person does generally.

Remind me often that I am loved

As I stated above, the low points in the life of a friend or loved one who has a depressive illness are definitely NOT the times for subtlety. This is a time when your friend or loved one who has a depressive illness needs to have things spelt out to them. Especially when they are wrapped in a cloak of darkness and feelings are involved. Love is most definitely the hardest one to understand from inside that headspace.

We have all had moments in our lives where we have felt unworthy of the love shown to us by the people who care. But for someone with a depressive illness it goes so much deeper than that, in periods of depression it can seem as though every little thing you do or say makes you less worthy of the love shown to you. It feels as though people have good cause to hate you for daring to breathe the air into your lungs, let alone anything real that you may or may not have done to cause harm or upset to those around you. It is very difficult to see the good in yourself, for the most part. Of course there are moments where this is not the case and you feel able to see positives but these are few and far between.

What YOU can do to help, is to ensure that you actually express love in verbal terms once in a while, don't expect that your friend or loved one who has a depressive illness to be capable of deciphering your loving actions as being such because when that veil is down it is all encompassing and they are just as likely to believe you hate them as they are that you love them, even if in general terms it should be obvious. Those three tiny words can mean everything to someone who is currently trapped in "everyone hates you land" say them often and never forget your love is a source of strength and courage when the road is hard.

Remind me often that you are there if I need to talk

When that veil of blackness is engulfing you, it is hard not to brush off offers of someone to talk to as being flippant and immediately assume that the person "is only saying that because it is what people say in this situation" rather than being a genuine and well-intentioned offer. If you remind your friend or loved one who has a depressive illness often enough then perhaps you will find that they somehow reach out to you and find it in themselves to actually hear your words as being true enough to take at face value. It is always a good thing to be reminded that you are not alone and that there is a hand awaiting you on the other side of the wall, if only you can bring yourself to reach for it. Remember though that sometimes, reaching for that hand takes all the strength and courage a person has left, so do your best to let them talk if they choose to come to you.

Ask outright if I am seeking advice or if I am just venting

It can be really difficult to talk to someone about your situation if they are prone to immediately offering an opinion or advice on what you should or shouldn't do. There are points in the cycle of depression where what you really need more than anything is to be allowed to empty your brain to someone. This is not because you need or even want advice, but because it is so full of everything and nothing that you cannot see past it clearly enough to think until you have spoken it aloud. When your friend or loved one who has a depressive illness sounds like they are venting out their frustration to you, it is totally ok to ask outright "would you like advice or do you just need to vent?" be sure to let them know that it is ok to have the time and space to just empty their brain, they will love you for it.

Often when a situation is bothering me, I know very well what it is that I need to do or say in order to resolve it, I just haven't realised yet that the answer to it is somewhere amidst the jumble of thoughts and emotions which are circling inside my head and talking to someone, even about something totally different really helps me to stop focusing on the situation for long enough that my brain has a eureka moment and suddenly I have a moment of clarity in which I discover that I do in fact know already the answer I am seeking. At that point even if someone told me in no uncertain terms what I needed to do or say I would not really understand it, until I have emptied the layers of chaos out enough that I can see it clearly and allow myself to consider it properly.

Sometimes I don't know the answers either.

There are times during the cycles of depression where a person is not sure themselves what can or cannot be a useful exercise in helping them to find the clarity they need in order to move forward. Knowing and accepting this will help you greatly in not getting frustrated with your friend or loved one who has a depressive illness. There have been many times when I have known very well that the support I needed was readily available, I was just unable to reach past the chaos in my head consciously enough to see what was before my very eyes. This is perfectly normal for someone who has depression and is not the person trying to be difficult, it simply is what it is, a period of indecision and inability caused by the illness which makes it increasingly difficult to look outwardly enough to see the avenue of change in thought or behaviour which is necessary for the situation to change enough that the person is able to begin recovering.

Keeping your word is more important than ever.

For someone battling a depressive illness, making plans to meet up with a friend or sharing some time with another person can feel like a big deal, if you are making plans to do something with a person in this situation it is very important to do your best not to cancel plans with them, as this increases their feelings of dissociation and can act as a barrier to them making plans with you in future. At the point in the depressive cycle where a person feels most vulnerable, they will already be struggling to control their brain weasels and things like saying you will do something for or with them and then not doing it are the kinds of thing which will contribute to making the person feel increasingly unwanted and like they are being bothersome when they really need something from you. Of course, it is not always possible to keep your word about things and I really am not saying that you should treat the person with kid gloves, the point I'm trying to make is that this kind of situation is the type of thing which can elicit a negative reaction from a person who is suffering from a depressive illness, because it gives food to the brain weasels and allows them yet another reason to attack the persons feelings of self worth or self esteem.

Do not behave in a flirtatious manner unless you mean it

During periods of depression it is hard to understand "everyday" behaviour of those around us, so if someone is being "play-flirty" with us it can be harder to distinguish whether they are actually being generous in their compliments or whether they are actually seriously flirting with us. There have been many times when the cloaks of depression have fallen that I have misinterpreted the behaviour of friends who have made "kind" comments and mistakenly taken them to be making some kind of advance.

When someone is in a period of depressive illness it is best to hold off on any kind of romantic advances until they are able to think more clearly. (Unless you are already in a relationship with that person, in which case disregard this section) This is because life inside the head of a person with a depressive illness is already very confusing; adding a new relationship into the mix generally only serves to make things more complicated.

Sometimes silence is the best thing to offer

Depression can make you feel as though you are the sole occupant of a desert island; although you can see and hear the outside world, your view is distorted, like looking through a patterned glass window. At times what you really want more than anything is just to "be" with someone; to spend time with someone during which your depression is NOT the sole topic of conversation. Don't misunderstand me, it is important to have opportunities to express the built up emotions which are locked inside, but it is equally important to have opportunities to feel like a normal human being too. After all, while depression doesn't necessarily go away forever, there are numerous periods of a person's life where depression is not the defining factor and the illness is under control, which allows life to return to normal.

All too often when I was at my worst, I would avoid people because those who I did see would constantly want to check up on my mental health, at the time what I longed for, but was incapable of seeking was just a couple of hours of "normal" where nothing triggering was said or happened, in the company of the people I loved. Of course, to them each day was normal, to me at the time each moment was spent battling my inner demons and simply trying to survive. This left me with very little energy to be able to even conceive the thought of asking for some company, let alone explain that I wanted to just "be" with them and not have to wear a particular "hat" or play a particular role in the moment. I wouldn't have known what to do with it back then, how to handle it or even what the social protocols were for such a situation. But in hindsight it would have helped a lot in terms of not feeling like I had failed at life.

Sometimes the person really needs your companionship more than your words of wisdom or advice. Depression is a lonely place and having someone to walk beside you; regardless of your communication abilities is a really positive and soul redeeming thing. In hindsight I wish I had tried harder to seek companionship when I was sick. It was incredibly difficult to find it within myself to spend time with those I loved because I was almost afraid that they would ask the questions that I did not know how to answer and I would feel honour-bound to be truthful, which would mean allowing myself to appear stupid in front of them for not knowing what it was that I was feeling inside.

Dad would come over and work in his den sometimes. although I would spend most of my time in my room, it felt good to have someone around, even though it rarely resulted in lengthy conversations, knowing that there was someone else about, with whom I could choose whether I stopped in for a chat or not was really helpful. It gave me the option of social interaction as and when I was able to chat. Often our chats ended in my sudden ranting, but his patience and kindness allowed me to let go of the shroud of my plastigrin sometimes and that really helped me to feel like I had an ally in those moments when I wasn't up to walking the few doors to visit with the family, it also allowed me the chance to talk to someone without fear of bumping into my little sister, from whom I was desperate to hide my illness. I was afraid that I would have to explain to someone who was too young and too empathic things that were, in my opinion far too big and complex for her to be capable of understanding. In hindsight I was incredibly selfish, though at the time I truly believed I was protecting her. Perhaps if I had stopped trying to hide from everyone I would have found myself better able to cope and seek the professional help I badly needed.

It is incredibly difficult to get someone who is in that situation to agree to spending time with another person. I would suggest trying to find activities which don't require much interaction but which allow the person feelings of companionship and the ability to just "be" without any pressure. Perhaps, get a copy of their favourite movie, some popcorn, ice cream and chocolate. Call a movie night. Be sure to tell your loved one that you don't care if they stink, are poorly dressed and you will not be offended if they scoff the entire tub of Ben and Jerry's. Explain that you want to hang out but you don't want to make them feel like they have to talk, so you'll bring a movie and there is no obligation to either watch it, or not to watch it. You simply want to spend some time together because you love them. Try to stick to this, as forcing them to talk will result in them running away from the situation.

What society as a whole forgets is that it is absolutely ok to simply hold space for a person, creating a safe environment for them without any expectation or necessity for discussion, but where that is also a perfectly acceptable thing to happen. We spend so much of our lives these days having fast, frantically paced interactions that it can difficult to just stop, sitting a while with someone, allowing silence or conversation, whichever is necessary or accessible at the time for the person. It is important to make sure that the person knows it is absolutely ok if they simply want to "be" and that you are totally prepared for that and will not judge them for needing silence as much as they need conversation.

This is especially important because in that headspace, everything you do or do not do can appear to be a cause for guilt, upset and ill-feeling.

I recall with sadness the amount of time I would spend avoiding my sister. I did not know how to explain to a child that I was trying to protect her from the monster that I had become; incapable of being the big sister she had come to know and love. So I hid from her. At the time it was my greatest source of guilt. I didn't know or understand how I could put into terms she would stand any chance of comprehending that every moment we shared felt like I was wading through treacle, trying to keep up a happy face for her sake, when what I really wanted to tell her was this "I love you more than anything, but right now I am really not feeling capable of being around you. But I want you to know, really know that you are my world, but I just can't be around you right now, I am too afraid that my presence in your life will have damaging consequences and that really is the very last thing I would ever want for you. So I am going to stay away from you for a while, not because I DON'T care, but because I love you more than life itself."

The truth is, at the time I was hiding behind her as my reason for not seeking help. In hindsight, as a role model to that wonderful little girl I should have taken my love for her and used it as a source of strength and courage, to stand up and say "I am not ok. I need help. I will get it for her sake". Sadly, hindsight is a bitter pill.

Time as a liquid

I have noticed over the course of my life that during periods of depression my sense of time changes drastically, minutes can take hours to pass and sometimes hours can pass in seconds without my really noticing. In the blackest moments time moves the slowest, whereas in my manic phases hours fly by faster than seconds. This can have a very detrimental effect on the mental health of the individual.

During deep bouts of depression it is most likely for me that minutes will seem like lifetimes. A conversation that is five minutes long can feel as though we have been speaking for months, partially because my brain is so busy taking note of everything and nothing all at once that the concept of time is lost within the whirlpool in my head.

I recall with pain the day that my foster mum took me to the gp because my medication was interacting and I lost control of my self harming to the point that I physically was not able to stop myself. Lunchtime at home was always 1pm. so it must have been just after 1.45 when my foster mum got the call to say I was in no fit state to care for myself and she came over. The doctor's appointment she made for me was at around 4 that afternoon. She barely left my side between those hours, leaving only long enough to use the bathroom or make tea. But those 3 hours felt like months.

Each second that I was left to my own devices felt as though she had been gone for hours. Yet the hours passed in just the very same 180 minutes that they would have any other time.

The worst thing about lacking any sense of time is that everyone who is outside of your head seems to think that time is a linear concept; it goes by minute by minute, day by day. But for the depressed person that is just not true.

Making plans for anything other than the immediate future (minutes or hours) can be absolutely torturous. Even when you know that something is happening in one week can feel as though you have years to wait. These moments can cause the brainweasels to throw a ball and leave the depressed person in a whirlpool of trying to understand something outside of their remit.

After moving to a new city in the middle of my deepest bout of depression I had to try to sort out my housing issues. So I went to the local housing office. It was a Friday and the man I spoke to asked me to come back on Monday with some paperwork. In reality it was two days in between, but for me those two days felt like 2 months. By the time Monday came around, I had completely given up on the idea of even returning to speak to him further.

My advice to anyone who is dealing with someone with depression is to be aware of this and try not to make the person plan too far ahead. The concept of tomorrow can be a difficult one to grasp in the darkness and organising anything for further away than a week often just exacerbates the person's feelings of hopelessness, depression and lack of self-worth. Having a diary which only makes the person plan a week, maybe two ahead can help the person not to feel overwhelmed by trying to understand the future.

Irritability

One of the most frustrating things about depressive illness is the fact that depressed people are irritable a lot of the time during periods of illness. The slightest thing can send you into a fit of feeling like the world is out to get you. It is incredibly difficult not to be angry at the people around you, partially out of frustration that the illness is making you behave strangely, forcing you to wear a veil of self-hatred that you can neither understand, nor explain and partially because it is suddenly inexplicably difficult to relate to the world outside of your head. This can result in you being snappy, generally moody and coming across as being aggressive, when what you believe you are doing is reacting perfectly reasonably to stimuli from the outside world. This can be extremely difficult both for the individual involved and for those around the person.

If you are aware that someone is dealing with a depressive illness, I would suggest that you firstly and most importantly don't take their irritability to heart. It is not really aimed at you, though by being the person standing in front of them you may well be the one who bears the brunt of their frustration.

Once you are aware that someone is not well mentally, try to realise that sometimes the person will be so busy hearing the negative automatic thoughts that it is almost impossible NOT to misconstrue your words and actions.

I recall when I was sick, pretty much every conversation I had with my parents would result in my going to my room believing that they hated me. Something as simple as "fancy a cuppa?" would be misconstrued as being "let's ask her a question she can't answer so she'll feel stupid" Of course in reality it was simply an offer of a cup of tea, but because I wasn't mentally up to thinking straight everything appeared inside my head as being a vendetta to prove to me how stupid/useless/worthless I was.

Therefore I would immediately reply with sarcasm, bitchiness or outright rudeness. Truly, it is one of those moments where if it were possible for you both to see inside the others head, you would both be laughing at the situation, but because that is not possible and things seem so gloomy to the friend or loved one who has a depressive illness, while appearing like they are simply causing trouble to the person dealing with them, it can be a source of unease and aggravation for all involved.

When these situations occur and arguments or misunderstandings erupt from them, either let it go and try not to take it to heart, or broach the subject gently and explain your side without proportioning blame. This can help to alleviate the potential of a repeat performance in the future.

A time for tears

Perhaps the hardest thing for someone who doesn't have depression to understand is that scary moment when the tears hit. I term it "scary" because in that moment you are hit with a plethora of emotions. There is a certain amount of fear because you find yourself asking "what if these tears never stop and I never manage to pull on my public face again?" This is often the very first thing to strike you when these particular tears hit. But on the flip side there is also a great deal of relief about their presence, as crying can help to release all kinds of tension, be it physical or mental. That said, (forgive me stating the obvious here, but I have known many people who thought this so I will spell it out) just because your friend or loved one who has a depressive illness has hit the crying phase does NOT mean that they are now magically fixed. It merely means they have reached the "crying stage". Often, there is nothing in particular that causes them; it's not like crying because your beloved pet just walked the rainbow bridge, or because your boyfriend just dumped you. These are tears which have good reason, but for a person who has a depressive illness tears are a double edged sword. Tears are the body taking the pressure cooker off the stove to release some of that built up pressure inside however it is impossible at times to know what exactly the trigger for them was and this serves only to make them more distressing.

If a friend or loved one who has a depressive illness lets you witness their tears, you should be aware that you are officially one of their VERY trusted people. I can count on the fingers of one hand the number of times in the ten years I have lived with depression that I have allowed someone to witness my "depression tears". That is not to say I haven't cried on the shoulder of a friend when my partners have dumped me or other "understandable" occasions. But depression tears are very much another story, they are the kind of tears where you feel utterly unjustified in crying because if someone dared to ask "what's wrong?" you would have absolutely no idea of the cause of your tears, so would be unable to explain even in the simplest terms and this can cause an incredible amount of guilt and feelings of stupidity.

During my worst depressive phase, the person I found myself turning to most often when the "depressive tears" hit was my dad. He never once asked "what is wrong? Why are you crying?" or seemed in the least uncomfortable with simply bearing witness to those moments. Often he would just allow me to vent out whatever was going on in my head, wait until I burned myself out, then offer hugs (always asking, never assuming I wanted or needed a hug) and reminding me that I was safe, supported and loved.

I would say that if someone has chosen to honour you by letting you bear witness to their depressive tears, there are some very helpful things you can do. Some of these things are obvious, but often they are subtle things which we don't always realise can mean something utterly different when your brain is wrapped in darkness.

When someone who is in the dark place starts to cry, don't immediately run to grab tissues as this can feel like a non-verbal "oh god, you're crying, what do I do?" signal, which can break the moment of openness and make the depressed person feel guilty for putting you into an uncomfortable position. This may sound a little weird, but in my experience, the handing out of the tissues has always felt like someone saying "dry your eyes, no more crying", this can prevent the person feeling comfortable with sharing these intimate moments with you in the future because from a depressed person's point of view, there's a level of guilt which makes you feel like you are an utterly horrible person for troubling someone with your issues, especially because these issues are often inexplicable in any tangible way.

It is incredibly important not to make the person who is confiding in you feel rushed or stupid for sharing these feelings with you. Often it is only the closest person who will even know there is a problem with someone who has a depressive illness.

This is mostly because of the stigmas attached to people with mental health issues. It can be incredibly difficult to come out and confess that there is something wrong which you are unable to explain in any tangible terms. You see, explaining that you are crying because suddenly your pot of "cope" has become empty and you have no idea what you are crying about makes you feel small and stupid,. I would say, once the tears have stopped, ask if there is anything that you can do to help on a practical level, offer suggestions...maybe make them a meal, writing a to-do list, help with talking to professionals, hand holding at appointments, moral support as well as literal support with day to day life. But don't pressurise the person into getting involved in anything they don't feel up to and be prepared, the person may not know themselves what you can do to help.

Difficulty communicating thoughts/ feelings

When trapped in the turbulent cycle of depression it can be incredibly difficult to successfully convey what you mean to those you love. In my case, I was wrapped in a constant cloak of fear, guilt and shame. I found it increasingly difficult to say the things that I was feeling. One of the very best things my close friends/ family did was to utilise every possible medium of communication. In my darkest hours I found it easiest to communicate in writing form, whether that is via Email or the more traditional letter. I also found that blogging about my situation made it feel less scary a place to be and helped me to make sense of my situation without anyone having to hear the things I wasn't sure how to word without causing upset.

I would suggest that anyone dealing with someone who is struggling to communicate their feelings verbally should offer practical and varied mediums. If someone is struggling to tell you verbally, they might find it easier to put their thoughts and or feelings into writing, this allows them the time and space to word things in a way that feels appropriate and which conveys what they mean more precisely than the flippancy and immediacy of verbal communication.

The hardest thing was knowing that what I really thought or felt and what I felt able to express without scaring people or causing hurt were two very different things. For example there were times I felt utterly worthless and I knew that if I voiced that to the people around me, they would immediately respond with words of comfort or love, which I found incredibly hard to handle (more on this in a later chapter) but if I wrote what I was feeling it gave me a chance to breathe before they replied and thus perhaps be in a better headspace and more able to take on board their words and support, it also allowed me to think through what I was trying to say and thus be more concise in how I worded things and that reduced my anxiety about communicating.

For me, the majority of my interactions with family members at the worst points of my depression were incredibly painful for both myself and the people involved. At the time I thought I was protecting my loved ones by trying to hide my depression, mostly by avoiding them (though I lived with them) I would spend hours in my room doing little more than trying to exist and hoping it would go away if I gave it enough time. This meant that I was getting very little social interaction and although this was self-implemented, it didn't by any means make it easy or really help the situation.

In hindsight most of my face to face interactions with my closest family members involved my poor attempts at reaching out and letting them know that I was still in there, somewhere amid the confused, scared and kaleidoscopic jumble of emotions. It was increasingly difficult to hold a conversation that didn't in some way involve my mental health, what I truly longed for was to have a conversation about something, anything that was "normal" but unfortunately that was increasingly impossible for me to instigate as I lost touch with the reality that others were living in.

Opportunities to release frustration

There have been many points in my journey with depression where I was so full of frustration that it was impossible to single out just one emotion at a time in order to try to understand my feelings. Over the course of many years I have discovered that it is really very important to find ways to release that frustration, as otherwise it festers and is demeaning to your self esteem. Sometimes simple things like taking some quiet time away from other people can give you the space to clear your head, but others you need to be allowed to release it physically. One good example was the battle of shrubulf Hitler; I'll let you meet him for yourself in the following passage.

"There was once a shrub in my foster- mum's garden. It was pretty in a way that only a shrub can be. It had brown branches and leaves as green as Jack himself. (With help) I've spent the last couple of days tearing him down so that we could plant "usefuls" in there; you know herbs and suchlike.

It was a battle which ended up being more like a personal journey into the bindings of my brain. I want to share my observations with those of you interested in my personal journey.

When I first began the battle of the shrub I was convinced I had faced down my demons and was now working towards pulling the patchwork that is me back together. Little did I realise as my dear old foster- mum handed me the axe that I was really on a personal journey into my own internalised anger.

Yesterday I set to work, axe in hand...really only intending to split the mahousive root cluster into more manageable pieces. Thwack! went the axe. Not hard enough, the axe bounced back without cutting anything at all.

I paused for a moment thinking "I'm not gonna be beaten by a shrub. I have an axe and shrub dear, you are to be compost!

I have long since learned how to focus and internalise anger for use at a more productive time. I had bags of the stuff...until Foster- mum gave me the axe and a get outta jail free on destruction. I took a deep breath and I summoned up the emotions of the past month. All those moments of anger, all those moments of fear and self-loathing left behind from my old life. I channelled the anger directly into the axe, summoning with it the full force of my self-hatred. THWACRACK! went the axe as it struck its target sure and true...I smacked the hell out of that poor shrub, not once seeing the shrub as itself and not really meaning to cause the shrub itself harm other than in so much as to make it removable.

I spent most of the afternoon smacking that shrub with the axe. I hadn't exactly realised how angry I was, nor how much I had internalised over the past few weeks.

But as that shrub went from it's original beautiful state through it's semi-obliteration right through to the moment I lifted it's final root-system with my bare hands and put it onto the compost heap, there was a change happening. A change I hadn't seen coming and hadn't for a moment even dared hope for.

With every axe-fall, every spadeful of dirt that I shifted so heartlessly and without care, I released a little more of my anger, frustration and self hatred.

I won...Shrubulf hitler is now on the compost heap.

 Thank you Shrubulf for your life and your death...and allowing your death to be a useful one. I send your memory best wishes!"

   Sometimes when you are trapped within layers of frustration, you don't even realise how much that internalised anger is bothering you until it hits you full in the face that you are not really "feeling" anything other than a big jumble of indistinguishable emotions.

As a druid, it is well known that we talk to all kinds of animal life and have a certain reverence for trees and plants too. There have been numerous times, when I was in a really negative place and have wanted to rant at someone without ever hearing their response where I have found myself talking to trees, the landscape and anything else that couldn't run away when it got bored. One of the best examples of this is the gooseberry bush in foster- mum's garden.

I first moved in with my foster parents at the end of April, it wasn't a hot summer but it was the summer that will stick in my memory forever. I had just moved halfway across England, having left a toxic and unstable home with my birth mother who had emotionally abused me for most of my life. I had no real "life skills" when I left her flat and I had no idea what would become of me. Kind friends (now the people I consider my foster ((and true)) family) took me in and taught me how to function as an adult. Those first few weeks preceding the shrubulf Hitler moment were incredibly stressful for us all. They were so kind and patient with me while I learned what it meant to have a family who loved you and treated you with respect. Yet I felt like there was so much I needed to say, so much bitterness that my birth mother was incapable of giving me the love I deserved but never received that I didn't feel able to share it with my new family. For those first few months I would spend hours sitting by the gooseberry bush, reconnecting with the land and getting to know this new and unventured territory that was now my life. One sunny May evening I found myself sitting by the gooseberry bush and words just started to fall from my mouth, words I didn't feel able to share with another living human being. I realised quite quickly that I was having a discussion with the gooseberry bush. I told it of my hopes, my fears, my sorrow and my joy in this new world. For months I would talk to the bush, never once considering it must have made me look quite insane to anyone else. But sometimes, words are not what we need, a safe space and a listener ARE. It's been almost two years since I saw Gerald (yes, I even named him) and there isn't a single time I pass a gooseberry bush without smiling at the fond memories of those times when I spoke so freely to him.

Of course I am not suggesting that everyone goes around having a chat to the local flora and fauna, some of them are rather shady fellows, but what I'm saying is that there is no shame whatsoever in talking to/at whoever or whatever you find the most comfortable to do so with whether that be human, animal or vegetable. The important thing is that you are expressing the emotions, not how you personally are most comfortable in doing so.

Partaking in creative exploits is also a very good and useful way of releasing stress and constructively expressing emotions. The truth is, you don't even have to be the next Picasso in order to create. Just the simple act of painting something, making something or spending some time in a nourishing environment can really help to release locked in emotions and allow you to begin thinking more clearly again. Art is a big part of my personal "mental health first aid kit" and has always seemed to do the trick.

Art was the turning-point in my major bout of depressive illness. I signed up to do an online art course when I was at my lowest. I think this journal entry explains best how it helped me to find firm ground again.

"I signed up a little over a week ago to do an art course...I signed up mostly because I'm unemployed, lonely and wishing I had the courage to get out there and meet people.

Picasso was an artist. As was Monet. I am merely me...I paint a bit, I do lots of creative stuff but I was questioning if I would dare call myself an artist. So in my depression-fuelled frame of mind I signed up for this E-course. I figured I might as well add another failure to my ever-growing list. So I signed up, believing deep down that I wouldn't even manage exercise one.

Saturday came and along came week 1's work and the tutorials. Yeah, I thought...I'll maybe try them. (Knowing damn well I wouldn't). An hour later, I found myself looking at them again. Well...nobody would know if I DID try them, would they? I picked up a pen....before I knew it...I had done the first exercise...and then some!

well the week progressed and I found myself posting my offerings daily in the group on facebook. Others were too. some were much better than mine. But I figured this wasn't about judging others, it was about doing the exercises. I kept going...

The end of week one arrived. I hadnt cried in a couple of days, I felt like perhaps a purpose was coming along...maybe. I was painting and drawing like it was the air in my lungs. A few of the other students in the group have been chatting with me, I feel like all of a sudden my artistic skills aren't so important as the journey that i'm on. This journey that has been beginning for me these past eight or nine months, this "brave new me" that I set out to find.

Well anyway, what I want to tell you is this...for months, i've been searching for the "real" me. The woman who I am comfortable with. She's been utterly elusive thus far. She doesn't return my calls, or answer my internal questions....I wasn't sure she even exists.

But...this course, "unearth you creative nature" it's called. well, I'm not sure it's my "creative nature" I've unearthed, but it is *something* It appears that what I've really found is something much, much deeper than I ever expected from a free Ecourse on the great interweb!

I'm gonna tell you what I have found this past 9 days.

This past nine days I have found a voice inside me. A voice I have come to recognise as that of a friend. A voice who sits there and holds my hand at 3am when I have a "great idea for a doodle" or a "let's knit something crazy" She knows my faults, she has lived with them in her secret castle for the past 28 years. She is the one who has been posting my work in the group. She is the one who named me "Artist" she is probably also the one who named me back in April when this journey began. You see I lost a lot this year in the journey, I have been to hell and back but I have survived it and more than that...much, much more than that I have found MYSELF! She kinda snuck in, when I wasn't looking and looked me in the eye, while saying "*insert my real name here* honey, you ARE an artist. You are confident.

You just need to hold my hand and breathe. I am you and you are me, we are one. We are the real you! Get out there and show the world the light in your heart! You can do this!"

I have found the real me. She is an artist and a creator and she will stand up in a room full of strangers in 2 weeks time and she will sing a song she wrote!

I have finally come to know myself after all this time and I am so very inspired. I want to inspire others.

With thanks and deep love to the wonderful Jani Franck and my fellow journeyers on the course. To each of you I send a large gift-wrapped box of self-belief!

I fully recommend the course, for details you can find it on www.janifranck.com

Yours always in love and light,"

As you can see, the darkness began lifting for me when I started to allow myself the time and space to create. Most of my early artwork was pretty rubbish if I'm honest, but it was never about the end result, it was always about that space in time where I was able to focus on everything and nothing all at once and not have to think in depth about anything that was bothering me.

To this day I often find myself going off to do art when I'm feeling stressed and it has become one of my most positive coping mechanisms. I would suggest that encouraging your friend or loved one to find an activity that they enjoy which allows them too freely and constructively express themselves is a very positive thing and should be one of the main tools in anyone's "coping toolkit".

Physical activities such as exercise or walking out in nature have also been great sources of frustration relief for me in the past. They allow your body to work off the excess energy in a way which is not harmful or negative. They also give useful access to vitamin D which helps to lift your mood and can help to alleviate some of the symptoms of illness.

Dealing with the manic phase

During my dealings with the dreaded black dog I have had periods of mania, which have occurred variously throughout my adult life at vastly differing levels of severity. These periods of mania can last anything from days up to months at a time and are very much a debilitating symptom of my depressive illness.

There are points in the illness where I reach a place emotionally where I am incapable of making healthy choices because suddenly I feel untouchable, as though nothing can possibly go wrong, regardless of the reality of the situation. This can often result in my becoming obsessed with a particular activity/hobby/thing and being incapable of stopping myself from making rash, badly informed decisions. Even if I recognise that I am in a manic phase, it can be extremely difficult to ground myself enough to prevent myself from ignoring rational brain and listening to absolutely excited cannot possibly see anything that could go wrong brain. This phase of manic episode reminds me of those infamous computer games of the 1990's featuring Mario and Luigi, mania for me is that moment when you have just been shrunk and nothing can harm you for a few seconds, except that it can be a permanent state for a few weeks. Obviously this is only the case inside my head, as reality just does not work like that, but this is the closest thing I can think of to explain to someone who doesn't experience this how it feels.

Two years ago I was signed off sick by my doctor from my job working as a carer in a residential care home. My boss was not terribly understanding about depression and thought I should be capable of turning it on and off at will. Obviously this is not the case and subsequently I was forced to resign or continue working nights which was negatively impacting on my mental health. The day I resigned (I was still far from thinking straight) I announced to my family that it would all be absolutely fine; I was going to start a business. I would start a mobile tuck shop selling all the bits and pieces that older people in care homes need but can't necessarily get hold of. Instead, I bought hundreds of pounds of card making materials and made frankly the ugliest cards possible. The more anyone asked about this big plan I had, the more I would enthuse to them about how utterly amazing things were and how I was really going to revolutionise care for the elderly by giving every home in a 50 mile radius access to this amazing service I planned to run. I ploughed not only money I didn't have, but literally every waking moment into these hand-crafted cards and I never had a clue why this tuck shop business wasn't working out and I wasn't getting rich from it! (I hadn't actually DONE anything about the idea. It was just a huge pipe dream. I literally *got as far as insuring myself and getting business cards done. Never actually *started* the business) I was broke. The more anyone tried to tell me I was heading for trouble, the more I assured them I knew very well what I was doing and would become irritable or explain that I had thought it all out. I was relying on my family to support me financially and yet, every penny in my pocket went straight out again on frivolous, pointless objects I would probably never use. By January 2013 (literally four months since leaving my job at the nursing home) I had run up £900 worth of debts and had no official address as life had become unbearable for my family and I was asked to leave. That is not to mention the money I owe my dad, for having bailed me out repeatedly from getting into these situations.*

By the time I paid off all my official debts they had risen to almost £2000. The threatening letters started to arrive. The bank, a mobile phone company and the insurance brokers threatened to take me to court repeatedly. Each time I got a letter I would look at it and say "oh dear. I'll deal with that tomorrow." I had a mountain of these letters. At times I was thankful when they arrived; it was almost a comfort to know that somebody still cared I was alive. Finally It reached a stage where one day I woke up and thought "oh my gods, what AM I doing? This is insane! You owe more money than you know what to do about. Everyone is tired

*of your ridiculous behaviour now sort yourself out!"
I went to the doctor and asked them to restart me
on the medication that the psychiatric team at
Swindon had recommended and started the ball
rolling in sorting out the mess I had caused. For a
few months I was paying them back a tiny bit each
week, as that was all I could afford. Then my luck
changed a little; a tax rebate came in which
covered all of my official debt and a small start
towards what I owed my parents, so I could start to
rebuild my life.*

It is often extremely difficult to get through to
someone who is in a state of mania with rational
concepts such as organising their finances in a
sensible way or producing some kind of business
plan. However it is possible, it simply takes a little
more thinking outside the box than usual.
Someone who has lived with the depression for a
while and is at a place where they are able to
recognise that they have different phases of the
illness are likely to be a lot more willing to listen to
your thoughts than someone who is going through
a manic phase for the first time, this by no means
says that it will be easier, simply that they may be
more willing to think about things twice.

I would suggest openly talking to them, offering
to help them to make a business plan and doing
your best to steer them in a sensible direction. But
at all times remember that YOU are not
responsible for that person's behaviour.

Sometimes they will not be in the right headspace to listen to your injection of common sense and may become aggravated with your input quite easily this is because inside their head their behaviour (however ridiculous it may seem to you) makes perfect sense to them. Catching the person in a moment of clarity will help to reduce both of your stress levels.

Try to refrain from criticising them openly, but try to offer suggestions which will help them to see a more sensible way forward for whatever they are attempting to achieve.

My aunt actually gave a great example the other day, I had recognised that I was behaving in a way which was conducive with mania, she simply said "aren't you getting a bit ahead of yourself with that? Would it not make more sense to start *here* instead?" it's a couple of simple questions, but ones which helped me to stop, take a step back and realise that I was jumping ahead way too far with the project I am working on. It did not feel as though she was being critical, thus I was able to take on board that I was jumping ahead so far that the project would not work out if I had taken that route without first setting the foundations of what I was trying to achieve. This really helped me to look at my own behaviour pattern and see the points where I was behaving in an irresponsible manner and gave me the opportunity to stop, think and reassess what I was trying to achieve.

In my experience I also find it extremely irritating during these stages of depression if someone tries to discuss or get me to think about something unrelated to whatever the thing is which I am obsessing about. This often comes out as hysterical behaviour such as yelling, crying or being verbally aggressive. This is because I am so consumed by the thing at hand that anything else lacks any kind of importance for the duration of that manic episode. I have discovered that what helps in this situation is to make a to-do list and ensure that it ends with say 20 minutes or an hour of whatever it is that I am obsessing about at the time. This ensures that I do whatever other chores or things are necessary before I run out of energy from solidly working on that thing. It can be difficult to instigate this kind of regime to a person who is obsessing, but it is very much a necessity, as it can help to reduce the feelings of mania and assist in a return to everyday life. This can also help to reinstate a healthier sleep pattern, as I have come to realise that in periods of extreme manic episode I lack the ability to switch off the activity which is my obsession for long enough to consider sleeping. The high level of energy means that I am capable of spending days without sleep while I plough all of my energy into doing the obsessive activity, to the point where I forget to eat or sleep. Therefore having some kind of set routine means that I have a cut-off point where I know I have to stop for the day, so it prevents my hyperactivity and potentially allows me to get some rest.

Relationship to exercise/ going outside

During the different stages of depression, it can be quite surprising how variable the person's energy levels are. Some days you are absolutely on par with your "normal" self, but others you can barely muster the energy to get out of bed, let alone consider exercise. Unfortunately, this is yet another of those utterly counterproductive situations. When you are experiencing low moods, exercise is one of the few things which are clinically proven to help lift said mood, via the release of endorphins. While it can be difficult to encourage someone with so little energy to get exercise, it is important to try to encourage them to live as "normal" a life as possible. The further a person recedes from the norms of life, the harder it can be to reintegrate into society once they are feeling better. It is far from a simple situation to remedy, but there are a number of things you can do to help.

Suggest going for a walk, or meeting for coffee somewhere. This will help to get the person out of their home; their four-walled prison, which will in turn lead to them having some sense of normality about their life. This feeling can be invaluable when you have spent days, weeks or even months trapped between those four walls it can end up making you feel as though you have cabin fever. Short outings help no end in raising mood levels and give an opportunity to clear the brain fog a little by offering a change of scenery and headspace.

Reading a book in the garden (weather permitting of course) can be a source of relaxation and a good way to get some fresh air.

Walk to the shops instead of taking the car, this gives them a sense of purpose which will mean they soon forget that they are exercising, but still get all of the benefits of fresh air.

Encourage them to do anything that takes their fancy (within reason) but try hard to get out into the world, as staying inside the whole time will really impact on their mental health and will not help at all with keeping them buoyant and giving you the strength to see through the darkness.

Relationship to food

When your brain is constantly mulling over reasons that you are worthless and that nobody cares one iota whether you live or die it can be difficult to remember to eat or drink. Inside the head of a friend or loved one who has a depressive illness who is not coping well with daily life, food truly is the first or last thing that they are able to think about. In general it goes one of two ways. I either binge eat all the wrong kinds of foods or I forget to eat at all. Often I fluctuate between the two for extended periods of time.

I recall when I was at my worst, the guys at the local takeaway (fried chicken was my binge-food at the time) knew me not only by name, but would know automatically what I was going to order without my giving any details at all. It got to the point I knew almost every delivery driver they had by name and would even ask after their families. At this point these people were the only ones I would communicate with willingly for days at a time, even then only out of necessity. Sure my two housemates were around and I would speak to them, but it truly wasn't out of choice at this point. I was swimming against the raging tide of trying to behave normally in the hope nobody would see the glaringly obvious. I was really not very well at all.

I also recall the carrots. They were in my fridge of months, never eaten, never really intended to be eaten. In hindsight they were purely decorative carrots which I could claim to keep stocked up on in order that nobody would realise I lived on a solid diet of fried chicken, ridiculous amounts of chocolate or nothing at all. My foster-mum would have KILLED me had she known the levels of rubbish I was eating. At times I would go days without eating much of anything, and then I would reach a point where my body would suddenly start craving something and force me to eat. At this point I would eat everything in sight; I could quite happily eat 10 pieces of fried chicken, a tub of ice cream and 3 portions of fries in one sitting.

What I would suggest for anyone who's loved one is in such a situation is to firstly attempt to limit the amount of unhealthy or fast food you keep in the house. Make small portions available for the days when "I'm not hungry" is the call of the day. Have fruit on offer often, as the sweetness acts as a temptation when there is no chocolate available.

It is also important to consider the preparation time of foods, as if something is hard to make or if preparing it will take a long time then this can act as a barrier to successfully making and eating it. I would say a food with a 10-15 minute preparation time and maybe 30 minutes cooking is much more likely to be eaten than something such as lasagna which takes a while to make fresh.

Try not to worry. I know it is a scary situation when someone you love is refusing to eat, (but under these circumstance) given time, they will get hungry. Try tempting them with smaller portions. A few mouthfuls at a time and don't overfill their plate as this can make the prospect of eating daunting to someone who hasn't been eating much.

Also if your loved one has been going through a self harming phase, do bear in mind that they may not feeling comfortable with having to use a knife. (I know this probably sounds ridiculous to you, but having been in that situation myself; I was terrified that it would be a temptation to cut myself. Especially when living/ eating alone). So serving food which can be eaten with or without a knife can also alleviate some of the stress surrounding meal times.

Sleep

Sleep is one of the many variables in the life of a person living with a depressive illness. At best, you have a reasonably normal sleep pattern like everyone else. At worst depression can leave you staring at the walls for hours on end, with your brain thinking up every possible way that you are the absolute worst person on the planet. The problem with depressive illness insomnia more so than regular insomnia is that you are already in that dark place in your head, where nothing you do or say is ever going to suffice and so when you are then sleep deprived on top of that, the world can seem so much bigger and more frightening.

For me I have two very different forms of insomnia, manic insomnia and exhaustive insomnia. The manic insomnia is when I am in a phase where everything seems utterly amazing and I am almost certain that I can fit a week's worth of hours into every day because "X project is just so utterly life changing and therefore absolutely MUST be finished right this very second" and thus I forget to sleep as my brain is over-filled with a blind excitement where I am incapable of seeing the destruction that I leave in my wake both to myself and others. Of course the problem with this kind of insomnia is that you don't even realise that you are utterly exhausted until your body finally just knocks you out, when you may well sleep for days as your body attempts to catch up on the sleep debt that you have unwittingly run up.

The exhaustive insomnia on the other hand is where the body is utterly exhausted and you are so unable to switch off your brain that you are unable to relax enough to even consider sleeping. This form is the worst. It is like giving four hundred of your greatest enemies each a spear and telling them "whenever you feel like it, go right ahead and stab me" except that each enemy is a mini-me of your own voice and the spears are utterly convincing statements about how little you are worth or how much of a burden you are upon society or those around you that you are simply unable to stop thinking for long enough to relax and go to sleep. The problem with these little warriors is that the more you lack sleep, the more believable their constant hate-speech becomes as you lay there, utterly frustrated and increasingly convinced that everyone in your life is out to get you or has some bizarre reason for hating you and yet being kind and loving to your face.

There are two main areas of sleeping problems, one is getting to sleep and the other is staying asleep.

Staying asleep when suffering from depression can be difficult. However, it is important to remember that during different levels of depression a person may need more or less sleep than normal, I know that during my mood lows, I often find myself sleeping much longer than I would during periods of wellness.

There are many factors to consider when it comes to finding ways to improve sleeping patterns. Firstly, it may well be that the illness is the main cause of the sleep problem and that can make it harder to change the situation. However, some things to consider are, whether the person is trying to sleep in an environment which is not conducive with the possibility for relaxation. This can make a big difference, especially if the person is trying to fall asleep in a noisy or uncomfortable environment.

The temperature of the bedroom can also make a big difference when it comes to the ability to relax enough to get good quality sleep. Ensuring that it is neither too hot nor too cold can really help to set up a place of relaxation and calm where sleep can come easier.

Ensuring that the bedroom is sufficiently dark enough can also help. I recall one place I stayed had a street light right outside my window and it was really hard for me to "switch off" my brain for long enough to get to sleep there. Using thicker curtains or adding blackout lining to the existing ones can help to create a less visually stimulating environment and thus allow a little more opportunity for sleep.

Small changes in a person's routine can often help. I have found in the past that making sure I am off of the computer an hour before I intend to sleep can assist in turning down the volume of my "daytime" thoughts and this allows "sleepy head" to take over. Therefore choosing to make that time "calm space" is useful. Avoiding drugs (non-medicines), caffeine, cigarettes and alcohol in that hour before bed also helps to reduce the levels of stimulation that the body receives in that "calm zone" and this also helps to reduce the "chemical stimulation" that often results from the ingestion of such substances.

If physical symptoms are the reason that your friend or loved one is struggling to get off to sleep I would suggest speaking to their GP and seeking medical advice, there are many things that the doctor is able to assist in reducing the symptoms of and therefore allowing more accessible sleep patterns.

Personal hygiene and cleanliness

During periods of depressive illness, it is my experience that one of the very first things to happen is the house becomes a mess. It is nothing new for me to realise that there isn't a single clean cup, knife, fork or plate in the house. This is because I am too busy conversing with the brain weasels to realise how much I have detached from what is going on outside of my head. This has become one of the first signs I look for during periods of my life where I am not fighting depressive illness, as noticing it allows me a chance to respond in the early days and potentially be able to make changes which may help to alleviate the symptoms and thus avoid a full blown depressive fit.

The way I deal with this when I notice, is first of all to stop and take stock of my emotional situation over the period of a couple of days, decide whether I have a "legitimate non-depression based" reason for whatever situation I am in, then move forward monitoring myself via either a mood diary or just generally keeping an eye on myself in terms of mood, energy level and relationship to food and drink. Once I feel ready to start the process of sorting things out, the first thing I do is to break the tasks necessary to clear up my living quarters down into smaller steps. Perhaps on the day in question I will wash up as much as I have energy to do. Then the next day clear all the rubbish...breaking the task down helps not to cause a burnout of energy but allows the task to be achieved. The truth of the matter is simple, it is not so much that the person is being lazy; it is simply that their worldview is skewed by illness and they are not really taking much notice of their surroundings.

I would suggest (as per the introducing normality section later) helping them to break down the tasks into more manageable chunks, if you live together, make the task simple such as you wash up and they dry and put away, or vice-versa. In the same way other tasks can be achieved.

Personal hygiene tends to be the other thing that gets overlooked. As you become more trapped in the internal world it becomes increasingly difficult to think about the "real" world. As a result the simplest of things such as maintaining personal hygiene get overlooked because they take more energy than you have in that moment. It is a tricky situation to deal with someone who is unwell and smells terrible but it is doable. Gently, but firmly tell the person "I don't mean to cause offence but you might want to consider a shower" as they probably won't actually have acknowledged this fact from inside their head. Try not to sound judgemental when you say this as the person is quite possibly utterly unaware that they smell terrible.

You see, the difficulty of dealing with chaos inside your head is that it has a bad habit of become chaos outside your head too. There are a number of things that you can do to help with both of these things. Firstly, be honest with the person about the situation, explain to them that you are not nagging, but are simply concerned for their welfare. Then help them to put into action a plan which does not feel too overwhelming to them, but which sets out clear, achievable goals. This not only helps them not to go into overdrive with trying to get things done all in one go and becoming frustrated when they fail, but also allows a sense of achievement in having completed the tasks required of them, raising their self-esteem and allowing a little space from the internal chaos which has engulfed their head.

Seeking professional help

When a person is dealing with a depressive illness, it feels absolutely counter-intuitive to seek professional help. This is because the illness does its best to convince the depressed person that they do not need or want help to get better, or rather that there is no hope of getting better. When you are staring into the blackness that is depression, it is extremely difficult to conceive the idea that there is someone out there who is capable of helping you to battle the illness and regain some control over your life.

The thought of seeking that person out is an incredibly difficult one to envisage, let alone find energy for. There were many times when I was not managing my depressive illness when the thought of telling someone "I'm not coping" was way beyond anything I could even begin to imagine. To consider seeking professional help was the one thing that truly scared me. Even more than the idea of ending my life.

You see, when someone is living inside the veils of depression it is hard not to become obsessed with words.

As a person who is battling depression you are constantly locked in a battle between rational thought and the dark, negative feelings which make you long to hit the self-destruct button. This means that on one level, the rational level you know that the things your brain is telling you cannot possibly be true, but this does not make them any less real or believable on other levels. So believing strongly enough that you are capable or deserving of the chance to get well can be hard. I was lucky, my foster-mum was amazingly helpful and sympathetic, allowing me the time and space to talk to her about things, but getting to the point where I would openly do so was hard going for us both. In that moment, any comment relating to your mental health feels like a well aimed insult and you feel trapped between the scary truth and hiding in a joyless ignorance.

During the lows of depression it is incredibly difficult to seek professional help because you are trapped in the bubble mentioned earlier in the book, where nothing outside of yourself quite seems to reach you. However, even though the bubble prevents you from communicating effectively on a receiving level, it is hard not to find yourself obsessing over words, which makes communicating your thoughts and feelings with someone outside of yourself, especially with a professional, it feels like their formality makes it even more important that you find the right words or phrases to explain your situation to them. At my worst I found it very difficult to explain anything relating to my illness to anyone.

In hindsight this is because I found myself tangled in a vast web of etymology of whatever concept I was trying to explain. The simplest of concepts became very difficult to explain because I would find myself worrying that I had not chosen the right words or phrases to best explain myself. Imagine going to visit the doctor to tell them you have a blister on your foot. Suddenly you are absolutely convinced that the blister will somehow offend the doctor if you mention its name. Now that you are incapable of saying "blister" then you decide to tell them "there is something wrong with my foot" but all of a sudden your ownership of said foot might also cause offence. Perhaps if you just said "there's something wrong with THIS foot" it would be ok...but what if they are now offended by your vagueness? (It goes on like this until you are so totally tied up in words, ownerships and confusion until seeking help seems like the single most ridiculous idea known to man)

The following sounds a little off the cuff, but it is in fact simply a description of what is happening inside the head of someone in that situation on a moment by moment basis during a doctors consultation, for your reference.

Eventually your friend/ family member has made the appointment for you and accompanies you to ensure you actually go to seek the help you need. You sit in front of the doctor and suddenly you are wondering whether you ought to compliment them *or something, you give banal responses to the questions, "I'm fine" and you automatically put on the plastic grin you use to cope. Anything akin to crying or truthful emotion would be an absolute disgrace. All of a sudden social grace is incredibly important, more so than telling them what is wrong. You say nothing. Not a word. Inside your head there's a conversation between yourself and the depression about all the reasons you should not tell them ANYTHING. "They are evil, they will put you into a straight jacket and cart you off to an institution" all manner of wild scenarios spring to mind. Eventually your loved one speaks on your behalf. You don't have the energy to make them stop, you hear them telling the *truth* of things, how you are pushing them away, behaving like a zombie, "not quite right", for a moment you hate them, they are helping the enemy, showing them your weakness but deep down you KNOW. You KNOW they are simply telling the truth. Shame envelopes you; suddenly you feel like you are wasting everybody's time and energy, you should give up. You should give in and let the illness win. But you can't because you are here now and arguing with your loved in front of "them" would serve only to show an emotion and that would be failure, your deepest fears engulf you and it feels like you are forced to watch as the world turns upside down. Finally you crack and tears begin to fall, words fall from your lips and you realise, you are speaking, telling them that you are not ok, that*

*you are not coping. They don't appear to be
reacting badly; on the contrary in fact, they seem
to be offering help. Your fear increases, what if this
is just another illusion? Does "help" really mean
help or is it a play to deceive you into falling
deeper into the blackness? You look into your
loved ones eyes, they seem to be reassuring you.
You realise that you haven't the energy to fight any
more, so you allow the doctor to do whatever it is
that they believe will help. In this moment you long
to feel safely cocooned in someone's arms but it is
impossible to seek out that safety because a hug
would hold too much honesty and you cannot bear
to let anyone see that deeply.*

I would suggest maybe running through with
your loved one the general "what will happen at
the appointment" to allow them some kind of
mental preparation as this will relieve at least
some of the stress and help them to not feel so
alienated at the appointment. Also offering to wait
in the waiting room helps too because sometimes
it can feel almost impossible to speak about
something as sensitive as depressive illness with a
loved one sitting beside you. This is because you
already feel ashamed about the situation and it
can feel as though telling the doctor some of your
deepest, blackest thoughts in front of someone
you care about is likely to cause that person to be
shocked or ashamed of you for even thinking half
of the things which have happened inside your
head. Know that this is not a judgement on you for

being there; it is simply the illness trying to segregate the ill person from their family and close friends because seeking help might mean getting better and that is absolutely not what the illness wants the person to do.

Advocating for loved ones

There are points in the cycle of depression where a person is incapable of advocating for themselves. This is the point where you may be needed to act as their voice to healthcare professionals and carers.

This can be a very awkward thing to do for someone in this situation, especially if they are trapped in the world inside their brain most of the time, as they may be incapable of understanding your viewpoint or disagree vehemently because they are unable to see the irrationality of their behaviour. The truth is, nobody likes having to confess that they are incapable of living a "normal" life. Society tells us that we must all be "strong, independent humans" but at times it is simply impossible to do so. The best course of action here is to explain to the person in need your reasons for concern and try not to take any resistance to heart, it is the illness they are angry and frustrated at, not you personally.

I recall at one point my medications were interacting with one another and resultantly I was very unstable for a while there. I was lucky; I have chosen family in healthcare professions, people whose opinions I respect, especially when it comes to my health. The particular day in question I had the foresight to contact aunty Karen and ask her advice as I was unable to stop self injuring and it was "out of character" knowing my usual patterns of self injury. I recall being so caught up in the veils of fear that I may use the wrong words to tell foster- mum what was happening and unintentionally cause her alarm and distress, that I got myself so frustrated that in the end Karen called my foster- mum, with my permission to ask her to come over to my house and support me in seeking the professional help I needed.

The day in question is mostly a blur even now, but I do recall quite clearly the way that my foster-mum took on the role of advocate between myself and the doctor that night. She had realised much earlier in the day that I was incapable of really expressing anything other than "I'm not well" so she took me to the doctor (mostly because I wouldn't have even got to the doctor without her there by my side, partially because leaving the house was a seemingly insurmountable task and partially because I wouldn't have had the first clue how to express my inner world to someone from the outside world who didn't know me particularly well.) At the appointment I was still unable to communicate my thoughts and feelings. What my foster- mum did was a perfect example of how to advocate for someone so I will share with you some bullet pointed suggestions here from what I recall she did/ said for me.

• Don't show shock or fear where possible as this just exacerbates the situation.

• Don't ask the mentally ill person to make difficult decisions at this point, it is too difficult to relate to the world, let alone think about it in logical terms.

• Ask the person if they would prefer for you to do "the talking"

• When speaking for them: state the case then ask the person "would you consider that a fair account of the situation? Or did I miss anything? Would you like to add anything?"- Sometimes having the pressure off to make sense of the main situation allows a little of the brain fog to clear enough that they can think of other useful information to add.

• Once your friend or loved one is starting to speak for themselves, offer to wait outside if that will help them to feel more comfortable in expressing their feelings to the professionals. (Sometimes it can be very difficult to explain a thought or feeling when someone you love is in earshot. Especially when it comes to mental health because being mentally ill is a scary enough experience without needing to consider the thoughts/feelings of people you love and have no intention of hurting/upsetting with the vitriolic voices inside your brain.)

Mental illness can be a lonely place. Don't forget to remind your loved one that you are on their side, the going just got tough, they need the reminder (and in actual words, not just in actions)

Depression is a lonely mistress, she will ensure that sufferers misinterpret other peoples actions so that only negative things get through, so stating blatantly the facts makes it a little easier to decipher and much less easy to misinterpret as meaning something quite the opposite of what you meant to portray.

Introducing some normality

After a long period of mental illness it can be inexplicably difficult to reintegrate to your usual routine and way of life. Partially this is due to people treating you as though you might explode at any given moment, but also because you have missed out on so much of their lives through being in hermit mode that it is hard to keep up with current events. During my worst journey through the blackness I missed out on so many of those little moments that families share, I grant you it was of my own doing but that never made it any easier to bear, nor was there an easy way to reintegrate without necessitating a discussion about what had come to pass. A conversation that I was in no way ready for, nor had I the right words to make amends.

There are many things that family and friends of people with mental illnesses can do to help a person to rediscover some semblance of normality in their lives and ultimately regain their independence and dignity.

Firstly I'd like to talk about routine as this is a big one for me personally. When I am out of routine for any length of time other than perhaps a couple of days, I find myself becoming much more anxious than when I know what I am supposed to be doing and when. I also find that having some kind of routine means that I remember to eat and sleep more appropriately than when I am just bumbling along with nothing in particular ahead of me. What really helps me is to have "set" mealtimes for main meals such as lunch and supper as this prevents me from ending up either starving, then bingeing on junk food or forgetting to eat altogether. It is especially useful because it means that I can also plan meals better if I have a routine as then I am able to shop more effectively and ensure that meals for myself are nutritious and well planned.

When I was at my worst, I was incapable of thinking even two steps ahead of where I was at the time; therefore it really helped me to have some kind of to-do list. The simpler the better, in terms of being specific as to what each task required as at this point my brain was so out of touch with reality that I would become confused easily and then get so side-tracked with the most bizarre things that nothing would get completed as I had gone off on a tangent of incomprehensible origin. What helped even more than that was to break said list down into smaller tasks, this made it seem much less daunting than a list which comprised of several seemingly unrelated things.

When your loved one is stuck in the veils of darkness, you could really help them by assisting in the formation of such a list and helping them to break it down into bite sized chunks. This not only helps to alleviate the overwhelming sensation of seeing a ten item list and thinking "oh Goodness, how on earth will I do all of these things? Where do I even begin? Oh no! I'm going to fail at this because it's all too complicated." But it also allows the person a sense of achievement when they realise that they have completed the list and this helps to raise their self esteem and prevents them from feeling further guilt caused by the alleged "failure".

Another thing which really helped me was having a single task which was my sole responsibility each day, a constant task, which made me feel like I had some kind of purpose. In my case it was the care and feeding of our pet chickens. There were three of them, they were called brownie and the ninja's but were very much kept as livestock (or so my foster- mum claimed until I named them and accidentally taught them that hugs are actually very nice) each day it was my responsibility to feed, water, collect the eggs and clean them out when necessary. This gave me a task which led to me building my own routines around it, however there was a very much unexpected development. Forgive me if I sound a little whacky here, but over those first couple of months, I found myself bonding with "the girls" and would often talk to them and even more often offer them hugs and affection.

There were many times when I was unable to find words for my human friends, but those chickens (who now live in my foster- mum's back yard) would listen, without ever passing judgement. In caring for them, I found myself learning how to be responsible for someone or something. There were a number of times in my suicidal days, when I found myself unable to end my life because of that unshakeable fear "foster-mum won't know I didn't feed them and nobody else knows the girls as well as I do. Brownie needs me alive, because nobody else gives her hugs" which I know, may sound a little crazy but in all seriousness, my responsibility to those girls helped me to maintain some kind of routine even in my darkest days. Also beneficial is the social interaction side of things. An animal doesn't expect you to make conversation, nor have the right words for any particular situation. You are a source of affection, food and shelter, the sole method communication is non-verbal; this doesn't mean it is not an entirely valuable form of communication, merely that it is much easier to relate to something in that headspace who cannot be offended by your wrong choice of words.

When assisting someone who has a depressive illness to organise themselves via a to-do list or routine, it is important to remember that the phases of depression have vastly different energy levels attached to them. Someone who is in the "crying" phase may have very little energy, as they are using up a lot of it in the outpouring of emotion, whereas someone who is in the mania phase may well seem to be attached to a mains electricity source. Therefore trying to have a mixture of labour intensive and less taxing tasks each day is often a good idea, especially if some of the more labour intensive tasks are able to be broken down into less daunting tasks.

During times of mental distress it can be surprisingly difficult to make a decision. There were times during my darkest hours where being asked "would you like tea or coffee?" seemed like an insurmountable question (regardless of the fact I rarely drink coffee). The very act of making a choice seemed to become increasingly difficult as my control over my mental health lessened. Suddenly I could think up four hundred possible outcomes of making the wrong choice. "If I choose coffee will that put the tea growers out of business? What if I was supposed to choose tea?" soon enough I would work myself into a frenzy of utterly overblown outcomes. Sometimes this would be delayed until the moments when I couldn't sleep where I would find myself discovering new and ever more complex ways that every economic problem on the planet was somehow connected to my making the wrong decision over what to eat or drink, do or say.

In hindsight the creativity with which my brain was working was impressive, but at the time it was impossible to stop working myself into the most pointless frenzies over things I couldn't possibly change.

At times like this I would suggest helping the person to make the decision by offering the least options possible, taking out the things you know for certain that they will not want. This can at least narrow the options and thus make the decision less daunting to make. As for the over-thinking, I would suggest simply explaining in a logical way the reality of the situation. You cannot stop the thought process for them, but you may be able to help the person to rationalise it, this may help to stop them from obsessing about the possibilities long enough for reality to kick in.

I will say before going any further that the last 2 chapters of this book are a potential trigger for feelings of self harm and for this reason I ask that you do not read these chapters if you feel at all unsafe at this point.

(They begin on the following page)

Self injury

One of the best known but most often misunderstood and stigmatised symptoms of depression is self-injury. Society as a whole seems to be under the impression that anyone who self injures is seeking some kind of attention or "special-ness" however I would like to dispel that myth right here and now.

There are many forms that self injury can take, some much more obvious than others, though in my case it has most often been cutting. Although I am not by any means saying it is the only form, this is the one I am going to cover in this chapter, as I certainly wouldn't feel comfortable, nor would it be right of me to try to discuss something of this gravity which I was not familiar with in enough depth to give useful advice.

Self Injury is one of the more frightening aspects of depression related illness. It can be just as scary for those around the person as it is for the person who is compelled to cause themselves harm.

Often when a person is self harming it is not about shocking or attention seeking from those around them, quite the opposite in fact, it is extremely rare that anyone has any idea that I am in a self-harming phase, unless they are in my close circle, in which case I may choose to confide in them that I am not doing so well at that point and that I am concerned as to my mental state because I have returned to unhealthy coping mechanisms.

Self harm tends to occur at the point in my depressive illness cycle when I have slipped down the mood slope to a point where I cannot begin to see a way back up, let alone choose to seek the help I need. Cutting becomes like scratching an itch, it's almost subconscious and for just a short while releases the pressure built up within my body.

I haven't cut myself in just over a year, as I have discovered other ways of releasing that build up of pressure and fear. For the most part, if I can find ways to distract myself, then I am able to remove myself from that headspace for a while and try to trust that the urges will pass. In my experience creative or artistic activities help to distract and allow expression of the kaleidoscope of emotions in some outward way, which helps relieve those feelings of pressure and isolation from the outside world.

One thing I would suggest to anyone dealing with someone who is self injuring is to leave the guilt-trips at home. The truth is, when someone is self-injuring they are not doing it to seek your attention or pity or to make you feel guilty, their self-injury is a reaction to their inner world. Something inside of them is making them feel like they need to inflict pain upon themselves, whether that is a reaction to pressure or a reaction to numbness. In depression there are many points where you feel absolutely nothing and are unable to make any correlation between the nothingness you feel and any kind of emotion whatsoever. (This is often a trigger for self-injury).

I think this entry from my personal journal explains best how it feels to let someone see your sites of self harm when you are in a place mentally where self-harm is your coping mechanism.

"Yesterday was one of the worst days I've had since I moved here. I am really, really not well and I reverted to cutting myself. I wasn't aware that my meds were interacting with one another and I was totally out of control. I hate to admit it, but in all honestly I scared myself half to death. I thought one little cut would release the pressure enough to put me back in control of myself, that nobody would ever have to know about it, I could pull on the plasti-grin and the world would be none the wiser. But it didn't help. It was like waving a red rag at a bull and after that first cut I couldn't stop myself. The more I tried to control the monster within, the more it insisted that I hurt myself, the more it pushed, the less resolve I had. Honestly, I have never felt so afraid in my life and I didn't know how to stop, or even what was triggering me. Right now, I'm half

convinced I should be locked up for my own safety.

There are 17 new cuts in all, the most I have ever done in one session and I feel at an utter loss in understanding what the hell has happened this past 24 hours.

Yesterday morning I got really scared and called Karen. Karen asked me to call foster-mum and get her over because I really wasn't well and Karen is like 250 miles away, so couldn't really do anything practical to help from there. I tried. I called foster- mum but ended up asking random questions about Emily coming over and found myself hiding behind the plasti-grin, making small talk as though there was no cause for alarm at all. I just couldn't do it. I couldn't find the words. I had no words to ask her help. All I had was a heavy veil of fear, shame and self-hatred which wouldn't let me say those words "foster- mum, I need you here. Now. Please come" Instead I called Karen back and told her I couldn't possibly bother foster- mum as she was busy. A couple of hours went by and I had been talking to Karen constantly, trying to keep myself busy, to hold on in the hope that my sanity would return. Then foster- mum called to say that my little sister and her friend wanted to come and play on the trampoline. I managed to maintain the plastigrin long enough to get foster- mum off the phone, then freaked out. I was terrified, what if [little sister's name] saw me, she would know immediately something was seriously wrong. I freaked. I went to my room and called Karen back; to ask her how best I could hide from them all. I half knew she wouldn't help me hide, but I couldn't face foster- mum and I certainly wasn't up to being a responsible adult for [little sister]. In the end Karen asked my permission to call foster- mum on my behalf. After much denial and attempting to convince her that I would manage alone, I caved in because I was terrified. It took everything I have to hand over the reins to her, to let her tell foster- mum; the one person who believed in me that I have finally proven my lack of worth. That I have gone back to the old way of handling things and that this time I am an absolute failure because I couldn't even stop myself.

Karen called foster- mum and sent her to me.

Foster- mum came over. Her first words to me were "Is there anything I should know?" I wanted to lie, to say anything other than "I've really lost it this time"...instead, I stared at the carpet as I pulled up my trouser leg to expose the semi fresh cuts which spanned the majority of my calf. I couldn't bear to meet her eye. I knew she must hate me now; must think of me as a disappointment and a failure. In that one moment where her gaze was drawn to those still bleeding cuts I felt it, it built and swirled like a venomous snake coiled and waiting in the very pit of my stomach. I felt so ashamed, so exposed. So naked. It was like being forced to walk down the high street with absolutely nothing on and having no choice but to expose the very core of who you are to the one person on the planet you respect and love more than anyone in order that you might live and then being expected to behave like nothing just happened. It was horrible knowing that she saw me so bare, so devoid of the plasti-grin, so ill and knowing it must now taint her very opinion of me.

Foster- mum on the other hand was great about it. She didn't bother with unnecessary questions and barely reacted outwardly, like this was an everyday occurrence. If I hadn't known better I would have said nothing changed between us, except it has, so very much changed in that moment. I caught fear in her eyes. Perhaps the problem is we know one another too well, I couldn't have hidden this from her in the same way she couldn't mask the flicker of fear in her eyes from me. My entire world crumbled and shattered before my eyes as the beautiful and wonderful woman I have spent months trying to prove myself to, got to finally see that I am little more than a burden to her and her family. I really hate myself right now. On an academic level I know this was a chemical reaction and therefore not really my fault, but deep down I just feel like I'm a failure who doesn't deserve a family. Let alone one as kind and loving as this one.

She took away everything sharp, just as I asked her to and never even batted an eyelid about doing so.(except she left R's knife block in the kitchen, little does she know that damn paring knife was the start of this whole mess. She'll never know that and I will never tell her.)

Right now I am scared, alone and feeling very much like I want to be far from here so I'll never have to face her again. Never have to be a source of her disappointment. If I asked, I know she'd be kind and gentle, but right now I would struggle to believe her opinion of me is anything other than that I am some kind of lunatic who should be kept away from the public."

Anyone who is supporting someone who has depression will know that it is an unpredictable illness which can warp any situation that you are in. Now I would like to state that my foster- mum has never judged me that was the illness speaking with its usual grasp of cold, hard, shame and fear. Depression needs you to remain too afraid to seek support or help; otherwise it risks losing its grip on you and having to allow you to recover.

Supporting someone who is a friend or loved one who has a depressive illness is a very difficult task and it is incredibly important for loved ones to know that the negative thoughts and feelings which the illness forces upon your loved one are absolutely no reflection of you in any way.

There are a number of other coping mechanisms, which are much healthier and/or much less damaging. Some of the self-harm prevention techniques which have worked for me in the past are the following.

• Distraction; losing myself in an angry game online, preferably war or strategy as these are the most involved kind of games and allow the venting of frustration without harming anyone in the physical world.

• Surfing the internet to distract myself.

• Using cognitive behavioural therapy techniques.

• When the urge to cut hits, holding ice cubes against my wrists as this simulates a pain response.

• Running my wrists under cold water.

• When I still have *some* control, setting myself a timer for half an hour and telling myself "if the urge is still there then, you can do it." Helps because usually the urges are gone by the time the timer goes off.

• Painting, reading, writing.

• Talking to a trusted friend about the situation. Preferably one that is not in the vicinity of me at the time, as this makes it feel a whole lot less awkward than talking to someone face to face.

• Writing a journal, somewhere private I can vent my thoughts or feelings without hurting anyone by saying the wrong thing.

Talking to someone who is in the mindset of self harm can feel very daunting and while I understand that the more comfortable response would be to avoid the subject altogether, it is necessary for you to offer the person the space to speak about it, however uncomfortable it is for you both at the time, it could well save their life later.

If my Aunt Karen had not previously known about my self-injury issues, I may well be dead now because I didn't know how to tell the people physically closest to me that things had got out of control. I thank the Gods every day that she had the courage to take that situation out of my hands. She probably saved my life that day and YOU could potentially save a life too. It really is as simple as listening, holding space for a person and allowing them to talk to you as deeply or as little as they are able or comfortable with doing so.

When discussing self harm, try not to show discomfort or alarm, instead listen and if you are unsure how to respond, it's quite simple. ASK. "What would help? How can I best support you in dealing with this? Is there anything I can do/ say?" but most importantly tell the person in simple terms "I am listening, I am here and I will support you as best I am able".

It is also important to mention here the possibility that when your friend or loved one with a depressive illness is trapped in that extreme headspace it may be necessary for you to take the decision that they are incapable of seeking help for themselves and seek that assistance on their behalf.

While on the whole I would hope that this would be a rare occurrence I will try to give some helpful pointers on what you can do in this situation.

Firstly, talk to the person, if it is clear they are not able to be rational enough to seek help for themselves, call their GP and make an appointment for them. Take them along and explain your concerns. Encourage them to speak freely and do your best to let anything negative they may say to or about you go over your head, chances are they don't mean it, it is the illness speaking.

Don't be afraid to seek support for yourself either, supporting a depressed person is an extremely difficult thing at times and there is no shame in getting yourself an arsenal of tools to make the situation easier.

Suicidal feelings/thoughts

There are points in the life of a person with depression when suicide seems like a viable option; an end to the pain and suffering that would make life easier for everyone involved. Obviously this is not truly the case to someone who's perception of the world is realistic.

There were many points during my deepest bout of depression where suicide seemed like a perfectly viable option. There were times where I would eat food with only a spoon because I was too afraid to trust myself with a knife. I was terrified of being left alone, but equally I was still determined to protect my family from the beast within me. All the while they still believed I had some kind of grip on reality I could lie to myself that I wasn't really as ill as deep down I knew I was.

At this point in my illness I was incapable of blogging my feelings as I was too out of touch with reality to be in any way capable of reaching out to the world. So I will try to explain how things felt from memory.

Mostly it felt like I was wading through treacle in a world to which I didn't belong. The simplest task was impossible because my creative brain would think up a hundred different ways that whatever I was holding/ using/thinking of could be used to end my life. The first time I considered suicide I had gone into Swindon to a job centre appointment (most of which I kept purely because I was afraid that my foster parents would realise something was horrifically wrong if I missed an appointment and the job centre called their landline). I recall looking up at the multi-storey car park across the road and thinking "I wonder how it feels to die falling from there. Actually that's a really easy way out. If I failed I could at least claim I was just looking over and slipped. Nobody would ever have to know that I had done it deliberately" I walked into the car park. The elevator was out of order. I walked up the first two ramps with a head full of nothing and everything at the same time, and then I ran out of energy, I slumped in a ball on the floor and cried. With sudden clarity I knew that I needed help, that I was no longer able to handle this myself. That my one true fear was startlingly close to becoming reality; someone having to break the news to my family that I had finally ended my life.

Even at home I was struggling to contain the bubble of self hatred that would engulf me. In the cupboard under the stairs was a length of rope, the blue kind you would use with tarpaulin or similar. For weeks I was locked in a private yet headlong battle with that length of rope. Each morning I would go and look at it, remind myself I wanted to get better and resolve to not let it kill me, it almost became a ritual, all the while it was still there, I could look at it and tell myself that it was an option when the time came. I found myself googling the most successful noose knots and how thick a piece of rope I would need to hold my weight. I realised quite quickly that if I couldn't source some then I could probably make use of the blue rope.

One morning I remember I was really out of it, the world had a sheen of sadness about it, something deeper than a thought, more an air of farewell and I knew that today would be the day I ended my life. I went to the bathroom, I got myself washed, dressed and prepared for my final farewell to this world. I went to the cupboard under the stairs, took out the rope and was just about to go into the garage when dad suddenly came in. On went the plasti-grin and suddenly I found myself pretending that this were nothing more than a normal day. His sudden appearance jolted me from the place in my head where suicide had seemed like such a good idea two minutes previously. He spent the morning in his den, right next to my bedroom. Periodically I would have to leave my room to go outside and smoke or use the bathroom. When I did it felt like I should make the effort to talk to him, even just to keep up the pretence of normality, I have always been a social beast, my silence now would have rung alarm bells, which would have forced me to tell him what was really going on inside my head. To this day he has no idea that in just those many little quiet conversations and moments where he allowed me to rant at him about random and various crimes that the people I loved had supposedly committed against me he saved my life. His presence in the house removed the opportunity for me to end my life without being discovered and thus prevented the illness from claiming another life for those few hours, by which time I had wrestled the beast within back to some form of quiet.

I would say one of the most valuable things you can do at that point is listen to the person. Try not to judge them. It is understandably a scary position to be in, both being the suicidal person and equally for a person who is dealing with someone who is having suicidal thoughts and/or feelings. The fact that they are talking to you about it is a very positive thing. Listening is incredibly important, reflecting back to the person what they have said to you helps to ensure strong communication between you. I would suggest not immediately talking to them about getting help, but instead let them talk, ask about what they are feeling, but ensure that your tone of voice is a non-judgemental one.

Do not leave them alone, at this moment they need to have someone with them at all times until the feelings have passed.

Once they have calmed down, then broach the subject of seeking help, Support them with finding out about services and sources of support in your area and do so together. This not only helps you to feel like you are doing something useful, but it also gives them a little more support to actually follow through on seeking that help. I know from experience how frightening it can be to have heard yourself say "I am suicidal" then have those around you trust you enough to seek the help you need alone.

Somewhere deep inside I knew very well that I would never find the courage to actually walk into the local mental health drop in centre and say "hi, I'm suicidal what should I do?" I was afraid, both of the consequences of admitting that to a mental health professional but also of what the next steps might be from there. I recall I stood outside of Swindon's "Mind" charity building for 45 minutes, I watched many people come and go, I smoked five cigarettes, each time I lit one I would say "right, after this one I will go in. Yes, one more ciggie and I will go in there. I am strong and I have courage" then I'd finish my cigarette and find any one of a thousand excuses not to knock on that door. After all, I didn't know anyone in there and I wouldn't have known where to begin in asking for help. An hour had now passed, I finally decided I could claim I had been, nobody would ever have a clue that I hadn't actually gone in there. I walked up the steps. I knocked on the door far too quietly for anyone to hear it. I waited about 10 seconds. Then I walked away. Now I could claim I had tried to seek help. I wasn't deliberately avoiding help and support, but I was far too afraid to knock on that door alone. I felt as though I had nobody left and no reason to bother trying to save my own life at this point, I wanted to die. I just hadn't figured out how best to achieve it yet.

For me it was very difficult to express to my loved ones that I had reached a point from which I felt there was no turning back. The opportunity to express myself to them was greatly diminished by my self-imposed exclusion from all family arrangements. My greatest fear was that my little sister would notice that the girl she knew and looked up to was actually gone and a rabid, vitriolic monster had taken her place. This meant that I avoided all meal-times with the family and would avoid any one to one time with foster- mum because I knew that she would see through the plasti-grin I plastered on in public. I was completely unaware that they all knew only too well that I was ill.

The truth is, at this point I probably would have benefitted greatly from being hospitalised and having the majority of my autonomy removed because I was unable to make rational decisions for myself.

As it happened I had realised that things were far from ok and was so afraid of myself that I took the decision to confide in my foster-mum and seek out the help that I so badly needed. I was lucky; I still had enough sanity to see that there was someone who could help me to get that help. Without her courage, strength and understanding I could not have even tried to get the help I so badly needed.

Note from the Author

Dear reader,

Firstly, thank you so very much for having read this book. It has been a hard journey delving into my own "ill-head" and pulling out the tidbits I have shared with you among these pages and I truly hope that they have given you some kind of insight into the things that go on inside the head of a depressed person.

When I began the journey of writing this book, it was only ever intended to be a personal thing I would give to my own friends or family that may perhaps help them to understand me a little better. But enthusiasm for my task blossomed and the book became what it is today.

If you have found even a little knowledge, comfort, help or understanding within these pages then the book has fulfilled my hope that my journey could help someone else along their path.

The journey through depressive illness is a long and hard one, the road has many ups and downs along its route and there are times we each face the scary prospect of giving up. My gift to you is a little wisdom I have learned along this road. While dark skies hover, there are always brighter ones head, true courage is holding on through the rainstorm and awaiting the kaleidoscopic skies of sunset.

Never ever give up hope, because without hope there is nothing left to hold on to. Under those darker skies, remember to reach out. Find what makes your heart sing and keep it in your arsenal of weapons against the brain weasels.

If you are supporting someone who has a depressive illness, then I thank you for giving that person a hand to hold in their darkness. Your role is hard and I really admire you for taking the time and effort to try to help someone.

If you are someone who has depression, hello fellow warriors, May the Gods bless you with limitless hope and a hand to hold on the journey. I won't tell you it will all be ok, because that is a cliché which drives me insane, but what I can and will tell you is that each experience you have with depression leads you to learning more about yourself and what works or doesn't work for you, with time and patience it does get easier to learn how to put in place ways which help you to function without everything being a trigger.

I want to thank everyone who supported this journey with kind words, support, encouragement, love and contributions to the Indiegogo campaign. The experiences shared with me by so many friends, family and even strangers that I randomly enthused at along the way were such an honour and I hope that the fruit of that journey can bless someone as much as I have been blessed by having you guys along for the ride.

In love always,
Alexis.

Useful numbers

ACTION ON DEPRESSION

Supports the running of self help support groups in various parts of Scotland which offer the opportunity for confidential local support and contact with others in a similar situation.

Provides an information service offering support and information on depression to individuals, their families and friends and professionals working with people who have depression; a quarterly member's newsletter and a range of helpful publications.

Telephone: 0808 802 2020 (free even from mobiles), Information Service, Wednesdays, 2:00pm-4:00pm

Email: info@actionondepression.org

Website: www.actionondepression.org

THE ASSOCIATION FOR POSTNATAL ILLNESS

The Association provides a telephone helpline. Information leaflets for sufferers and healthcare professionals as well as a network of volunteers, (telephone and postal), who have themselves experienced postnatal illness.

Helpline: 020 7386 0868, Monday, Wednesday, Friday, 10:00am-2:00pm and Tuesday and Thursday, 10:00am-5:00pm (national rate)

Email: info@apni.org

Website: www.apni.org

BIPOLAR UK (Previously called MDF - The Bipolar Organisation.)

A user-led charity that works to enable people affected by bipolar disorder (manic depression) to take control of their lives. Provides information, and a wide range of support services for members. Also helps people by supporting self-management, and with a national helpline and local self help groups throughout the UK.

Helpline: 0845 634 0540, Monday-Friday, 10:00am-4:00pm (lo-call rate)

Email: mdf@mdf.org.uk

Website: www.mdf.org.uk

DEPRESSION ALLIANCE

Supports people with experience of depression through a pen-friend scheme, membership and newsletter. Provides information and publications and campaigns to raise awareness of depression. Also operates a network of local self help groups throughout the UK, with support for new groups and information about existing groups.

Telephone: 0845 123 23 20 (to request an information pack only)

Email: information@depressionalliance.org

Website: www.depressionalliance.org

JOURNEYS

Journeys (Towards Recovery from Depression) is the only organisation with the sole purpose of supporting people affected by depression in Wales, and their family and friends.

Journeys takes a holistic approach to overcoming depression through guided self help, building the foundations for sustainable and long-term well being. Provides information, practical resources, services and training that promote the development of skills and strategies to help people find their own route to recovery, and also co-ordinates a network of self help groups.

Telephone: 029 2069 2891

Email: info@journeysonline.org.uk

Website: www.journeysonline.org.uk

SEASONAL AFFECTIVE DISORDER ASSOCIATION (SADA)

Information and membership packs for people effected by Seasonal Affective Disorder (also generally known as winter depression).

Website: www.sada.org.uk